THE HEART AND EXERCISE: A PRACTICAL GUIDE FOR THE CLINICIAN

THE HEART AND EXERCISE: A PRACTICAL GUIDE FOR THE CLINICIAN

Randal J. Thomas, M.D., M.S.
Assistant Professor
Department of Preventive Medicine
Department of Medicine (Cardiology)
Northwestern University Medical School
Co-Medical Director
Cardiovascular Rehabilitation Program
Northwestern Memorial Hospital
Chicago, Illinois

IGAKU–SHOIN NEW YORK • TOKYO

Published and distributed by

IGAKU-SHOIN Medical Publishers, Inc.
One Madison Avenue, New York, New York 10010

IGAKU-SHOIN Ltd.,
5-24-3 Hongo, Bunkyo-ku, Tokyo 113-91

Library of Congress Cataloging-in-Publication Data

The heart and exercise: a practical guide for the clinician/Randal J. Thomas, editor.
p. cm.
Includes bibliographical references and index.
ISBN 0-89640-302-5. — ISBN 4-260-14302-6
1. Heart—Diseases—Exercise therapy. I. Thomas, Randal J.
[DNLM: 1. Cardiovascular Diseases—rehabilitation. 2. Exercise Therapy. 3. Exercise. WG 166 H436 1996]
RC684. E9H43 1996
616.1′2062—dc20
DNLM/DLC
for Library of Congress 95-32008
CIP

ISBN: 0-89640-302-5 (New York)
ISBN: 4-260-14302-6 (Tokyo)

Printed and bound in the U.S.A.
10 9 8 7 6 5 4 3 2 1

To my parents, Claude and Bonnie Thomas;
To my wife, Jodee;
To my children, Erica, Natalie, Heather, Joshua, and Nicole;
To my teachers;
To God;
For making life happen in their own unique way.
With them every burden is lighter
And every joy grows deeper.

ACKNOWLEDGMENTS

The contributions of numerous people are gratefully acknowledged. These include the working groups from the 26th Bethesda Conference: Recommendations for Determining Eligibility for Competition in Athletes with Cardiovascular Abnormalities, whose important work guided our efforts in compiling this book. Gene Kearn of Igaku-Shoin Publishers, Inc., was a constant, patient, and insightful adviser. Rita Chabot, the production editor at Igaku-Shoin, helped put the finishing touches on the book with precision and wisdom. Finally, I thank my wife for her support and inspiration.

FOREWORD

My interest in the athlete's heart and in the cardiovascular benefits of exercise stems from my own athletic background. Physical training always made me feel better and generally made me function better as well, both physically and mentally.

I became interested in cardiac rehabilitation as a medicine resident at the Mayo Clinic in 1966. As a research project, we designed an exercise program for patients with angina pectoris, mainly to see if it would help enhance development of coronary collaterals. It did not, but the patients in the program seemed to thrive, uplifted by being treated as athletes once again rather than as patient-invalids. The Mayo program exists today, nearly 30 years later, and served as a template for our program at the Georgia Baptist outpatient cardiac rehabilitation program in Atlanta. Now virtually every major hospital in the city has its own program.

One of my role models was Dr. Paul Dudley White, who had a career-long interest in the athlete's heart and in the merits of physical fitness. His advice to former President Dwight D. Eisenhower to resume walking, golf, and other forms of exercise after his heart attack helped pave the way for a return of cardiac patients to the active lifestyle.

As early as the 1920s, Dr. White was advocating the importance of regular exercise and preventive medicine. In a lecture to the U.S. Public Health personnel, he said:

> You can all do something towards keeping your hearts and arteries in good condition. Most of you are careless of health even though you are intelligent in other matters . . .
>
> Exercise to keep fit. To be indolent physically is worse than to be excessively athletic; there is a happy mean . . .
>
> Use your arms and legs more, and your stomachs and automobiles less.

My work includes preparticipation screening examinations of college athletes (at Georgia Tech) and professional baseball players (Atlanta Braves), among others, counseling patients about the benefits, risks, and techniques of exercise and attempting to restore cardiac patients to optimal performance. In helping to organize medical care for the 1996 Olympic Games, I have been reminded of how much is known about the effects of exercise on the heart and other organs. All too often, however, the complexity and enormity of that information makes exercise counseling difficult for the clinician to implement in everyday practice.

I welcome this book as an up-to-date, authoritative guide that will help bridge the gap between what is known about exercise and what is implemented in practice. I know it will be a very useful resource for physicians and other health care personnel who deal with exercise counseling. I think it will also stimulate a quest for additional understanding of the fascinating interplay of exercise and the cardiovascular system.

John D. Cantwell, M.D.
Chief Medical Officer
1996 Olympic Games

PREFACE

Each day millions of Americans develop the goal of exercising, to get into better shape. Each day, unfortunately, fewer than half of them achieve that goal. Numerous barriers are blamed—not enough time, too expensive, not enjoyable, no place to exercise, or no one with whom to exercise. These barriers are well known to physicians, for we constantly deal with them as we encourage patients to exercise. We also deal with them in our personal struggles to keep physically fit.

Some patients have health problems that keep them from initiating or maintaining a regular exercise program. What we have learned from the chronically ill patients who surmount the barriers to participate in regular exercise programs (e.g., cardiac rehabilitation) is that exercise can be safe and beneficial to many people with health limitations. Unfortunately, we as physicians are not trained in methods to apply the beneficial effects of exercise therapy to the lives of our chronically ill patients. Even if we have learned the basic principles of exercise prescription, we generally lack the ability to "make it happen" for our patients.

From published data, it is clear that Americans are deficient in regular physical activity, as well as in exercise advice from their physicians. This book has been designed to help clinicians do their part in alleviating both problems.

Randal J. Thomas, M.D., M.S.

CONTRIBUTORS

Karen J. Calfas, Ph.D.
Chief Psychologist, Project PACE
Adjunct Professor of Psychology
San Diego State University
San Diego, California

John D. Cantwell, M.D.
Medical Director
1996 Summer Olympics
Preventive Medicine Center
Georgia Baptist Medical Center
Atlanta, Georgia

Mary C. Fahrenbach, M.D.
Fellow, Division of Cardiovascular Medicine
University of Massachusetts Medical Center
Worcester, Massachusetts

Carl Foster, Ph.D.
Program Director, Cardiac Rehabilitation
Milwaukee Heart Institute
Sinai Samaritan Hospital
Milwaukee, Wisconsin

David L. Herbert, J.D.
Partner, Herbert, Benson and Scott
Vice President
Medical Risk Management Services, Inc.
Canton, Ohio

William G. Herbert, Ph.D., FACSM
Professor
Division of Health and Physical Education
Director, Cardiac and Intervention Center
Director, Laboratory for Health and Exercise Sciences
Virginia Polytechnic Institute and State University
Blacksburg, Virginia

Barbara Long, M.D.
Chief Physician, Project PACE
Chief, Primary Care Sports-medicine, Student Health Services
San Diego State University
San Diego, California

Marla A. Mendelson, M.D.
Assistant Professor
Department of Medicine (Cardiology)
Medical Director
Adult Congenital Heart Disease Center
Northwestern University Medical School
Chicago, Illinois

Todd D. Miller, M.D.
Associate Professor of Medicine
Mayo Medical School
Consultant, Cardiovascular Diseases
Mayo Clinic
Rochester, Minnesota

Kevin Patrick, M.D., M.S.
Director, Project PACE
Associate Clinical Professor of Family and Preventive Medicine
University of California, San Diego
Adjunct Professor of Public Health
San Diego State University
San Diego, California

Jeffrey Roitman, Ed.D.
Assistant Clinical Professor
Department of Medicine
University of Missouri–Kansas City
School of Medicine
Director, Cardiac Rehabilitation
Heartwise Research Medical Center
Kansas City, Missouri

James F. Sallis, Ph.D.
Co-Director, Project PACE
Associate Professor of Psychology
San Diego State University
San Diego, California

Randal J. Thomas, M.D., M.S.
Assistant Professor
Department of Preventive Medicine
Department of Medicine (Cardiology)
Northwestern University Medical School
Co-Medical Director
Cardiovascular Rehabilitation Program
Northwestern Memorial Hospital
Chicago, Illinois

CONTENTS

◆ CHAPTER ONE ◆

INTRODUCTION: PROMOTING EXERCISE IN CLINICAL PRACTICE

Randal J. Thomas, M.D., M.S.

CASE EXAMPLE

Patient History and Examination

The patient, J.F., is a 55-year-old lawyer who sees you in your office 2 weeks after having suffered a myocardial infarction. His diabetic father died at age 60 of a myocardial infarction, and J.F. wants to know what he can do to prevent this from happening to him. He is concerned about the health of his heart and about the fact that he is overweight. He is also concerned because a physician in the hospital told him that he had borderline diabetes as well as borderline hypertension. J.F. has frequently resolved to begin a regular exercise program but has been unable to make time in his busy schedule to do so. In fact, he has not followed a regular exercise program since before entering law school more than 30 years ago. He does not smoke. His diet is unrestricted, and he currently exercises only about once a month when he plays a round of golf, using an electric cart. His physical examination is unremarkable except for a blood pressure of 148/92 and the fact that he is moderately overweight (31.0 kg/m^2). His fasting blood glucose level is 120 mg/dl.

Comments/Questions

This case example illustrates several important dilemmas, discussed in this book, that clinicians face as they evaluate a wide variety of patient-athletes. Among the questions considered covered in this chapter are: What are the specific benefits and risks of exercise?; What makes people want to begin and maintain an exercise program?; and Is there evidence that the clinician can help the patient-athlete begin and maintain a safe, beneficial exercise program?

INTRODUCTION: WHO EXERCISES?

It is not uncommon for clinicians to be asked by their patients for advice about exercise. At times, the patient is a sedentary individual with a gradually expanding waistline and an increasing risk of cardiovascular disease. At other times, the patient is a competitive athlete with a potentially dangerous cardiovascular condition who seeks your advice regarding the safety of athletic participation. Regular physical activity offers health benefits and some risks for nearly everyone, but who among out patient-athletes exercises regularly? Do national trends suggest that in the future more and more of our patient-athletes will be exercising regularly?

For more than 10 years, the U.S. Public Health Service has promoted physical fitness as one of the 15 areas of greatest importance in improving public health.[1,2] Still, reports suggest that the majority of people are physically inactive. For example, the Year 2000 goals for the nation's health include the goal of reducing the percentage of sedentary adults to 15%.[2] According to 1993 national data, however, the percentage of sedentary adults remains 24%, unchanged for the past 5 years.[3] The high prevalence of physical inactivity is even more dramatic among certain population subgroups, such as minorities and people of low socioeconomic status.[4,5] The percentage of persons with cardiovascular disease who are sedentary is thought to be at least as high as the percentage among the general population and is likely to be even higher. Among children and adolescents, there is evidence of a decline in both physical activity and physical fitness over the past decade. Physical activity has been reported to be particularly low among adolescent girls.[6] In addition, most schools have begun cutting back on organized physical education to the point where only 36% of children in grades 1 through 12 are enrolled in daily physical education classes. Even then, classes are often short and involve very low intensity physical activities.[7] If childhood physical activity habits carry over into adulthood, as most researchers believe, current trends suggest that adults of the future will be *less* active than those today. Clearly, new methods of promoting physical activity are needed.

Despite these discouraging facts, there is some good news: the percentage of physically active adults has increased gradually over the past 30 years. Although there are methodologic concerns regarding the strength and accuracy of this evidence, [8–10] more recent data, collected in a standardized fashion in 26 states between 1986 and 1990, support this finding.[11] These data suggest that since 1986 physical activity patterns have improved in two ways. First, slightly fewer adults are considered sedentary (completely inactive). Second, more adults are exercising intensively (at least three times a week for at least 20 min at a time of 60% of maximum exercise capacity or greater). Improvements in physical activity patterns have been particularly striking for women and the elderly (see Table 1-1). For instance, the percentage of women exercising intensively increased from 5.9% in 1986 to 9.2% in 1990 in women of all ages. A sedentary lifestyle decreased among all women, dropping from 34.3% in 1986 to 32.3% in 1990, although the majority of improvement was in women over age 55.

In contrast to women, men had generally less marked improvement in exercise patterns. Among men, for instance, the percentage of the population exercising

TABLE 1-1. Prevalence of physical activity patterns in various U.S. adult subgroups, 1986 and 1990, taken from the Behavioral Risk Factor Surveillance System from 26 states.

Group	Sedentary (1986)	Sedentary (1990)	Regular, Intensive Physical Activity (1986)	Regular, Intensive Physical Activity (1990)
Women	34.3%	32.3%*	5.9%	9.2%*
18–29	25.2%	25.8%	3.7%	5.4%*
30–44	30.6%	29.4%	4.4%	6.7%*
45–54	35.4%	33.4%	7.7%	13.4%*
55–64	41.1%	35.2%*	9.5%	13.8%*
65+	47.3%	42.9%*	7.7%	11.4%*
Men	31.2%	28.6%*	8.2%	9.0%
18–29	23.4%	19.3%*	6.6%	6.6%
30–44	28.9%	28.1%	7.1%	6.6%
45–54	39.3%	36.8%	7.9%	8.3%
55–64	37.1%	33.7%	11.5%	13.8%
65+	39.5%	35.6%	11.3%	16.1%*
Whites	31.5%	29.0%*	7.4%	9.9%*
Nonwhites	39.9%	39.5%	4.7%	4.9%
Non-high school graduate	50.6%	51.5%	4.2%	4.6%
High school graduate	35.3%	33.9%	5.3%	6.9%*
Some college	26.0%	23.6%	7.2%	10.3%*
College graduate	21.4%	17.9%	11.9%	14.3%*

*$p < 0.05$ for the difference between 1986 and 1990 figures.
Source: Adapted from Ref. 11.

intensively rose only slightly, from 8.2% in 1986 to 9.0% in 1990. Only men above age 65 showed a statistically significant increase in intensive, regular exercise (11.3% in 1986 compared with 16.1% in 1990). A decrease in sedentary lifestyle, on the other hand, was noted only in men below age 30.

These and other data from Caspersen and Merritt[11] are summarized in Table 1-1 and suggest several other interesting trends. First, as people age, they tend to polarize with regard to physical activity patterns. That is, the prevalence of both a sedentary lifestyle *and* intensive exercise increases with age, suggesting that people tend to become either very active or very sedentary as they age. Second, the improvements in physical activity patterns have been most dramatic among people over age 65. Third, some subgroups of the population show no significant improvement in physical activity patterns (e.g., nonwhites, low-education groups, and men younger than age 65). In fact, from 1986 to 1990 there was a slight increase in the percentage of sedentary adults among those who had less than a high school education (50.6% in 1986 compared with 51.5% in 1990). The most troubling findings from these data are that despite definite improvements in physical activity patterns among some subgroups of the population, only a minority of adults now engage in habitual physical activity.

Another trend in the United States and other countries that will impact on the clinical practice of medicine is the aging of the population. In the United States it is estimated that, because of increased longevity, decreased infant mortality, and decreasing birth rates, the percentage of the population who are over age 65 will increase from the current 13% to approximately 21% in the year 2030 and to nearly 24% in 2080.[12] If these predictions hold true, patients who visit clinicians in the future will be older and will thus be at higher risk of cardiovascular and musculoskeletal disorders than the patient of today. Consequently, patients of the future may require a more careful preparticipation evaluation and exercise prescription than the patients of today.

WHY DO PEOPLE EXERCISE? FACTORS AFFECTING EXERCISE ADOPTION AND ADHERENCE

Perhaps one of the most critical questions that all potential patient-athletes must consider is "Why exercise?". What prompts some people to exercise? What keeps others from doing the same? Clearly, these issues are central to any efforts we as physicians make in advising our patients to exercise, for these are the issues that help translate advice, desires, and resolutions into actions. Patient-athletes who visit clinicians generally fall into one of three categories: (1) those who exercise regularly, (2) those who exercise sporadically, and (3) those who are sedentary. These exercise behaviors, like many other health-related behaviors, are the result of a series of complex personal processes that are internal as well as external, both perceived and unperceived. Researchers have attempted to identify factors which influence exercise behaviors in the hope that such information can identify ways to motivate people to initiate and/or maintain a program of regular physical activity. Several factors (determinants) which influence the adoption and maintenance of regular exercise have been identified, and theories of behavioral modification related to exercise behaviors have been explored.

Determinants of Physical Activity

Personal characteristics that are associated with successful initiation of regular exercise include (1) male sex, (2) young age, (3) confidence in one's ability to exercise ("self-efficacy"), and (4) health consciousness (not smoking, eating a healthy diet).[13–16] Environmental factors that have been reported to help promote the initiation and maintenance of an exercise program include (1) a recommendation by a physician to exercise, (2) family support, (3) friends' support, and (4) accessibility of exercise resources (walking/jogging path, gymnasium, swimming pool, etc.).[13,15,17] The determinants of *adopting* exercise behaviors differ somewhat from determinants of *maintaining* those behaviors, however (see Table 1-2). For example, age, sex, perceived barriers, and self-efficacy for exercise behaviors are all predictors of exercise behavior *adoption*.[48] Frequency of injury and illness, attitudes toward exercise, moderate-intensity activities, and social support, on the other hand, tend to be good predictors of persons who will maintain an exercise program.[15,16,18]

Data suggest that more than 50% of individuals who begin an exercise program will either give up entirely or continue only sporadically.[19] Most people who fail to continue their exercise program do so during the first 3 months, as is the case with other health-related behaviors, such as smoking and alcohol use.[20] Longer-term compliance with exercise programs is relatively unstudied but is undoubtedly lower than in the short term.[19,21,22]

Basic Principles of Behavior Changes

Psychological theory and research have led to a greater understanding of the complex, dynamic mechanisms of behavior change as they relate to exercise initiation and adherence. Among the theories which have been suggested to explain behavior change, the *transtheoretical model* is well accepted and applicable to the clinical practice of medicine.[23–27] This model suggests that people move in and out

TABLE 1-2. Predictors of exercise initiation and maintenance

Predictors of Exercise Initiation	Predictors of Exercise Maintenance
Young age	Low frequency of injuries and illnesses
Male sex	Positive attitude toward exercise
Self-confidence in ability to exercise	Moderate-intensity physical activities
Health conscious (nonsmoker, good diet)	Family and peer support
Family support	Moderately high socioeconomic status
Friends with whom to exercise	
Recommendation from a physician	
Moderately high socioeconomic status	

of different *stages of change* in which they are more or less receptive to the idea of ceasing high-risk health behaviors or adopting beneficial health behaviors, such as exercise.[23,28,29] As described in Chapter 3, these stages include *precontemplation* (not intending to make a change), *contemplation* (considering a change), and *action* (actively engaging in behavior change). This model also suggests that people use various strategies or *processes of change* to move through the many stages of change. Some of these are interpersonal (e.g., identifying personal barriers to exercise) and others are environmental (e.g., finding a friend or family member with whom to exercise). Chapter 3 describes the PACE system, which helps clinicians identify patients' particular stage of change with regard to their exercise behavior. The system also provides practical suggestions to help identify the processes of change, which can be of help in attaining and maintaining the action stage of exercise behavior.

Two processes which are important in the dynamics of exercise behavior are *decision balancing* and *skill building*. The decision balance is the process by which a person weighs the pros and cons of a particular behavior change.[30] This process helps the person identify the incentives as well as the barriers to adopting the behavior in question. As would be expected, this balance tends to be influenced by the person's current stage of change. For example, individuals in the action stage tend to give greater weight to the positive aspects of a behavior change, while those in the precontemplation stage tend to give greater weight to the negative aspects.

Skill building is the process of focusing on the adoption of specific skills which will reinforce the person's efforts to change a health behavior (time management skills, for example). As the skills are developed, the person gains greater confidence (self-efficacy) in his or her ability to carry out the desired behavior. Consequently, behavior change is enhanced.[31–34] In one study, for example, self-efficacy in performing exercise was found to increase in post–myocardial infarction patients following a treadmill exercise test. This increase in self-efficacy predicted compliance with a prescribed exercise program better than the actual treadmill performance itself.[35]

BENEFITS AND RISKS OF PHYSICAL ACTIVITY

In Healthy Persons

As mentioned earlier, the pros and cons of exercise behavior are important influences on a patient's decision to begin or continue with an exercise program. When asked why they exercise, most patient-athletes give two reasons: (1) exercise provides immediate short-term benefits ("I feel better," "I like to compete," etc.), or (2) exercise promotes long-term health benefits ("I want to keep my weight under control," "I want to deep my heart healthy," etc.). While short-term benefits may have greater weight for patient-athletes, it is the long-term benefits which have been more widely studied (see Table 1-3). The health benefits of long-term, habitual physical activity, in fact, are well documented and include improvements

TABLE 1-3. Benefits of habitual physical activity in apparently healthy people and in patients with CVD

Benefits	Apparently Healthy People	People with CVD
Improved cardiopulmonary fitness	Yes	Yes
Decreased cardiovascular morbidity rates	Yes	Probably not
Decreased cardiovascular mortality rates	Yes	Yes
Decreased all-cause mortality rates	Yes	Probably
Lowered blood pressure	Yes	Yes
Improved lipid profile (↓ LDL and/or ↑ HDL)	Yes	Yes
Improved glucose metabolism and probable prevention of diabetes	Yes	Yes
Improved body composition (↓ fat mass and/or ↑ muscle mass)	Yes	Yes
Improved thrombolysis: thrombogenesis profile	Yes	Probably
Decreased cancer mortality rates (colon, lung, and breast?)	Yes	Probably
Improved psychosocial well-being (quality of life)	Probably	Probably
Enhanced return to work after cardiac event	—	Possibly
Protection against osteoporosis	Yes	Probably

in both physiologic and psychological parameters.[1] In addition, observational studies have consistently found that higher levels of physical activity and greater cardiopulmonary fitness are associated with reductions in all-cause mortality, morbidity, and mortality from cardiovascular diseases and morbidity and mortality from various types of cancer.[36–43] Physiologic improvements from habitual physical activity include positive effects on oxygen consumption and utilization, blood pressure, blood cholesterol, body mass, blood clotting factors, and heart rate.[44–46] Significant improvements in cardiac efficiency have also been documented following regular physical activity (see Chapter 2). Psychological improvements are less well characterized but appear to include favorable effects on mood and reduction in depression and anxiety.[47] Conversely, the health risks of habitual physical *inactivity* are significant and have been well documented. In 1986, in fact, an estimated 205,254 deaths associated with coronary heart disease (CHD) were attributed to never or irregularly engaging in physical activity. This number exceeds the number of deaths from CHD attributable to smoking (148,879), obesity (190,456), and hypertension (171,121).[48]

Several issues regarding the clinical benefits of regular physical activity are described below. These issues have particular relevance for many patients who visit their physicians for exercise advice.

EXERCISE AND BLOOD PRESSURE

Numerous investigators have studied the association between exercise and blood pressure. Much of the interest in this area focuses on the potential blood pressure–lowering effects of regular physical activity. That habitual exercise can lower blood pressure has been established by several lines of evidence in both hypertensive and normotensive individuals.[49] Individuals who are physically active have significantly lower systolic and diastolic blood pressure levels than their less active peers.[50,51] Harvard alumni who did not engage in vigorous exercise were at 35% greater risk of developing hypertension than those who did exercise, independent of other potentially confounding factors such as body mass index (BME) and a family history of hypertension.[52] This beneficial effect of exercise probably results from down regulation of the adrenergic drive and subsequent lowering of peripheral vascular resistance, heart rate, and blood pressure due to both acute and chronic adaptations to physical activity [53–55] (see Chapter 2).

Intervention studies have found that endurance exercise (i.e., walking, running, swimming) had more of a blood pressure–lowering effect than resistance exercise (i.e., weight training),[56,57] probably due, at least in part, to the increase in peripheral vascular resistance that occurs during resistance training. In addition to the type of exercise, the intensity of exercise is thought to determine the blood pressure–lowering effect of the activity, with low- to moderate-intensity exercise having as much or even more of an effect than high-intensity activities.[56,57] In one study, in fact, low-intensity exercise was found to decrease diastolic blood pressure significantly even though it produced no significant changes in maximal oxygen consumption.[57] Daily bouts of exercise lasting for at least 30 min have been reported to be more effective in lowering blood pressure than shorter, less frequent exercise regimens.[53] The blood pressure decrease observed in most exercise interventions had been 5–10 mm Hg for both systolic and diastolic blood pressures.[53,56,57]

EXERCISE AND LIPIDS

Observational and interventional studies of exercise and blood lipid levels suggest that their relationship is somewhat similar to the relationship between exercise and blood pressure. Like blood pressure, blood lipids show both acute and chronic adaptations to physical activity.[58] Unlike blood pressure, however, blood lipids change most remarkably with larger amounts and higher intensities of exercise.[59] Little or no change occurs in blood lipids when physical activity levels are below 1000 kcal/week; maximal improvements occur when physical activity is approximately 4500 kcal/week. For most patient-athletes, levels of physical activity may not be great enough to promote significant changes in blood lipid levels.[60,61]

Changes in lipids after habitual exercise have been reported to be different in women and men. For men, the major lipid change associated with exercise is a small to moderate increase in HDL cholesterol (particularly HDL subfraction 2).[59,62] In women, small decreases in total cholesterol and triglycerides have been reported.[59]

EXERCISE AND GLUCOSE METABOLISM

Evidence suggests that physical activity plays a key role in helping to regulate glucose metabolism through insulin-related and non-insulin-related mechanisms.[63] Habitual physical activity, in fact, may prevent or retard the onset of non-insulin-dependent diabetes mellitus.[64] The blood pressure–lowering effect of exercise is of particular importance for persons who have impaired glucose tolerance or diabetes, since the prevalence of concomitant hypertension is high in such people.[65]

EXERCISE AND BODY COMPOSITION

Many studies have explored the association between exercise and body composition. Results of these studies are mixed. In one study, for example, home-based, moderate-intensity exercise promoted significant improvements in physical activity and exercise capacity, along with a significant weight loss (1.5 kg).[60] Another, larger trial with a similar design found similar improvements in activity and fitness levels bout found no changes in body weight or body composition (body fat).[61] Part of the inconsistency in these studies may be due to unmeasured factors, such as changes in dietary habits, which may have confounded the potential effects of exercise on body composition.

Several studies, however, suggest that physical activity may play a key role in the regulation of body fat and weight.[66,67] Physical activity may, in fact, be one of the keys in treating the so-called Syndrome X since it has the potential to improve all of its component conditions (central obesity, insulin resistance, hypertension, and dyslipidemia).[68] It is important to remind patients that regular physical activity can promote important improvements in body composition even when it does not significantly decrease body weight. This is because habitual exercises can decrease fat mass while at the same time increasing lean body mass (muscle).[69]

OTHER HEALTH BENEFITS OF HABITUAL EXERCISE

Several other benefits of regular exercise have been reported. For instance, fibrinogen, a risk factor for cardiovascular disease, has been found to be lower among people who exercise regularly.[70] Plasma volume increases with regular physical activity, producing a reduction in blood viscosity.[71] These hematologic changes, as well as the possible increase in fibrinolytic activity of the blood after regular physical activity,[72] may explain part of the protective effect of exercise against CVD.

Several reports support the protective effect of exercise against lung cancer and colon cancer, as well as possibly protective effect against breast cancer.[73,74] Habitual weight-bearing exercise has been reported to delay the onset on osteoporosis in postmenopausal women. The evidence is somewhat mixed regarding the beneficial psychological effects of exercise, although consistent data suggest that exercise can reduce anxiety and depression.[75] The effects of regular exercise on the immune system are also uncertain, but research suggests that chronic exercise can improve immune function (e.g., natural killer cell activity) over the long term.[76] Exercise during an acute infection, however, may actually weaken immune function.

RISKS OF PHYSICAL ACTIVITY IN HEALTHY PERSONS

Serious cardiovascular complications of exercise are rare among apparently healthy people. Still, research has demonstrated that the risk of myocardial infarction does increase during acute bouts of exercise, particularly for people who are not accustomed to exercising regularly.[77] In fact, the risk of myocardial infarction during exercise is nearly 50 times higher in a sedentary person than in someone who exercises regularly. As described in Chapters 4 and 5, the absolute risk of exercise-related cardiac death is low among persons over age 35 and is even lower among persons below age 35.

By far the most common risk of regular exercise is the risk of musculoskeletal injuries. It is well documented that the greater the exercise duration, frequency, and intensity, the greater the risk of musculoskeletal injury.[78] In one study involving male soldiers who underwent 12 weeks of intense physical training, nearly 40% suffered training-related musculoskeletal injuries such as sprains, muscle stains, and overuse injuries to the knees.[79] Injuries were most common among soldiers who smoked, were previously sedentary, had previous injuries, and were older.

In Persons with Cardiovascular Disease

For years it was thought that physical activity was harmful to persons with preexisting CVD. However, researchers in the field of cardiovascular rehabilitation have found clear evidence of the benefits of regular physical activity for such patients. As described above and in Chapter 2, there are definite cardiovascular adaptations to exercise that optimize cardiac efficiency and improve several physiologic parameters that are critical to the patient with CVD. There is also growing evidence that higher levels of physical activity and physical fitness are associated with improvements in CVD and with decreases in all-cause mortality in persons with preexisting CVD. Several meta-analyses and reviews have consistently found that participation in organized physical activity programs (cardiac rehabilitation programs) reduces long-term all-cause mortality by approximately 20% among individuals recovering from myocardial infarction.[36–43] Organized cardiovascular rehabilitation begins during the first week of hospitalization (Phase I), during the intensive early outpatient period (Phase II, weeks 2–36), and finally during the maintenance phase (Phase III) , which continues indefinitely. Many low-risk patients (those without inducible ischemia, left ventricular dysfunction, or dangerous dysrhythmias) can exercise safely at home if given the proper instructions and follow-up by the clinician and his or her ancillary team.

In addition to reducing cardiovascular morbidity and mortality, exercise in persons with CVD appears to improve the physiologic parameters mentioned in earlier sections. Patients with CVD who exercise regularly also appear to improve their subjective rating quality of life, at least soon after a cardiac event,[80] and may return to work earlier than those who don't exercise following myocardial infarction, although this latter issue is still unsettled.[81] Exercise has also been reported to protect against noncardiac atherosclerotic disease, such as peripheral artery occlusive disease (PAOD).[82] Furthermore, exercise therapy has been found to dramatically improve functional capacity and quality of life in persons with PAOD.[83]

To the surprise of many clinicians and patients, the risks of regular physical activity are quite low for the majority of patients with CVD. Among high-risk individuals, of course, the risks of physical activity can be substantial, but for most patients who are of low to moderate risk, exercise can be safely undertaken if proper exercise prescription guidelines are followed (see Chapters 6 and 7). Several studies have found that, among participants in cardiac rehabilitation programs, serious cardiovascular events are rare, occurring approximately every 60,000–100,000 patient-hours of exercise.[84,95] No reports of musculoskeletal injuries or other health risks have been reported in people with CVD who exercise, but such risks are thought to be similar for apparently healthy people of similar age.

Benefits, Risks, and Intensity of Exercise: How Much Is Enough?

As alluded to above, the intensity or amount of habitual physical activity that is necessary to produce health benefits varies, depending on the benefit in question. For instance, lipid changes, cardiopulmonary fitness, and life expectancy increase in a curvilinear fashion with increasing intensities or amounts of habitual physical activity. Other benefits, such as blood pressure changes, body composition changes, and changes in psychosocial well-being, appear to be greatest for low to moderate levels of exercise intensity. What, then, is the optimal intensity or amount of exercise for patients? Clearly, the answer to this question varies from patient to patient, but generally speaking, low- to moderate-intensity physical activities provide an optimal balance between health benefits and health risks (e.g., musculoskeletal trauma, sudden cardiac death, and heat injuries). In addition, exercise program adherence is greater in low- to moderate-intensity activities than in high-intensity activities (see Appendix 2 for a list of physical activities by the intensity of energy demand). Figure 1-1 depicts the relationship between exercise intensity and exercise benefits, risks, and adherence.

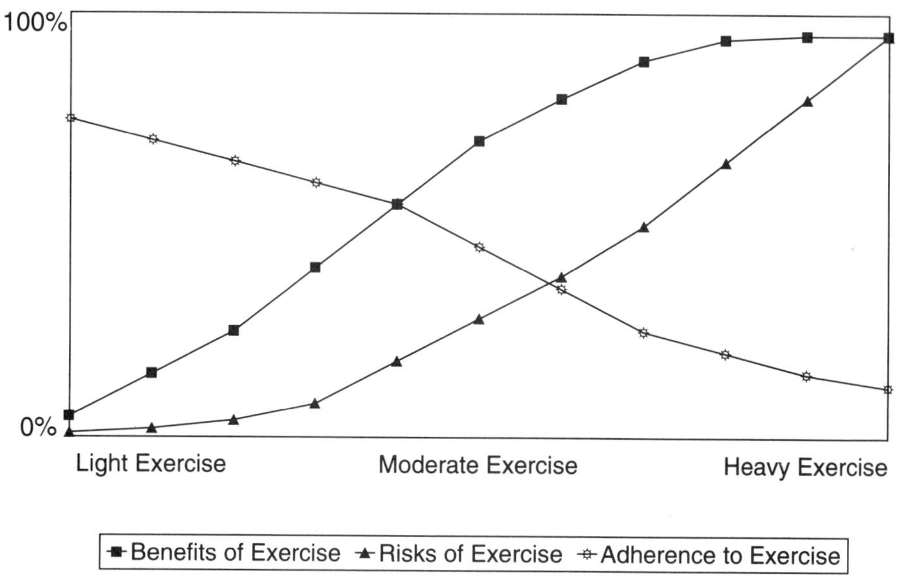

FIGURE 1-1. The relationship between amount of physical activity and associated benefits, risks, and patient adherence. For most people, low to moderate amounts of physical activity are associated with the optimal combination of these factors (i.e., maximized benefits and patient adherence with minimal risks). This relationship will vary for some patient-athletes who have greater potential benefits from physical activity (e.g., professional athletes) or greater potential risks (e.g., persons with symptomatic CVD).

PUTTING IT ALL TOGETHER: THE ROLE OF THE CLINICIAN

The knowledge of most physicians regarding the principles of preparticipation evaluation of patient-athletes and the prescription of effective exercise programs is usually quite limited. Nevertheless, patients often look to their physicians for expert advice regarding the nuances of exercise medicine. Most physicians lack formal training in exercise medicine, and even those who have such training usually gain it from sporadic individual study and/or personal experience on the athletic field. A small number of physicians have formal fellowship training in sports medicine. However, even for the well-trained and committed physician, making time to prescribe exercise for patients is often problematic.[86] In addition to lack of training, as described further in Chapter 3, physicians have several impediments to giving exercise advice, including lack of confidence, lace of reimbursement, and confusion regarding the specifics of the exercise programs. It is no wonder that only a minority of physicians consistently give exercise advice to their patients.[87,88] When the patient has cardiovascular disease, physicians may be even less inclined to give exercise advice, probably at least in part because the exercise prescription is perceived to be complex and potentially dangerous to such patients.

The average adult in the United States visits a physician approximately five times each year, generally for management of one or more chronic conditions, such as hypertension, diabetes, hypercholesterolemia, or obesity.[89] Many of these conditions, ironically, have direct and indirect associations with physical inactivity. Physicians, therefore, are in an excellent position to help their patients prevent or reverse adverse medical conditions by promoting and facilitating regular physical activity. In today's increasingly cost-conscious medical world, the attractive cost-benefit ratio of regular physical activity is of particular importance to clinicians as well as to patients.

In studies of other health behaviors, physicians have been shown to be able to provide simple, yet effective encouragement to adopt healthier lifestyles.[90] A few, generally positive studies have involved clinicians in counseling apparently healthy patients to initiate and maintain a regular exercise regimen.[91] Physician extenders have been successful in effectively prescribing exercise for persons with CVD.[92] Some surveys suggest that a large percentage of people would increase (or try to increase) their level of exercise if they were so advised by their personal physicians.[13] If a method can be developed to promote exercise that would be simple enough to be carried out in a busy clinician's office and yet remain effective, this would be a practical and cost-effective way to improve the public health of our nation. It is hoped that new methods, such as the physician-based assessment and counseling for exercise (PACE) method described in Chapter 3, can help busy clinicians carry out the critical work of providing exercise advice to their patient-athletes.

SUMMARY

1. Research suggests that the majority of U.S. adults do not exercise on a regular basis and that few school children are participating in regular physical activity

classes. Despite these negative facts, trends over the past decade suggest that there has been a gradual, slight increase in the percentage of adults who exercise intensively, particularly among women and the elderly.

2. Several personal and environmental characteristics are associated with an increased likelihood of a person's beginning and maintaining an exercise program. Among these, self-confidence, social support, and physician advice to exercise are of particular importance.
3. Behavior change is thought to occur as people move in and out of various stages of change (i.e., precontemplation, contemplation, and action). Various processes of change, such as decision balancing and skill building, can be used to promote movement of patients from one stage of change to another.
4. Numerous health benefits of regular physical activity have been documented, including improvements in cardiopulmonary function, decreases in cardiovascular and all-cause mortality, and improvements in blood pressure, blood lipids, glucose metabolism, and body composition. Similar benefits are attainable for apparently healthy patient-athletes, as well as for those with CVD.
5. Musculoskeletal injuries are common among exercisers, particularly those who were previously sedentary and those who exercise at high levels of duration, frequency, and intensity. Cardiovascular risks of exercise are low for most patients with CVD, and are even lower for apparently healthy persons. Still, careful preparticipation screening is essential to identify patients with potentially high-risk medical conditions that would make exercise dangerous.
6. Clinicians are in an ideal position to provide important and effective advice to their patients regarding exercise. Relatively few clinicians currently give such advice because of various impediments, such as lack of training, lack of time, lack of confidence, and lack of reimbursement. New methods, such as the PACE method described in Chapter 3, have been designed to make exercise prescription simple, safe, and effective in the hands of a clinician and his or her support staff.

REFERENCES

1. *Healthy People: The Surgeon General's Report on Health Promotion and Disease Prevention.*(Pub. No. 79-55071A) 1979, Washington D.C.: U.S. Public Health Service, Department of Health, Education, and Welfare, 1979.
2. *Healthy People 2000. National Health Promotion and Disease Prevention Objectives.* D.H.H.S. Pub. No. (PHS) 91-50213. Washington, D.C.: U.S. Public Health Service, Department of Health, Education, and Welfare.
3. McGinnis JM, Lee PR: Healthy people 2000 at mid decade. *JAMA* 273:1123–1129, 1985.
4. Shoenborn CA: Health habits of U.S. adults, 1985. *Public Health Rep.* 101:571–580, 1986.
5. Stephens R, Jacobs DR, White CC: A descriptive epidemiology of leisure-time physical activity. *Public Health Rep* 100:147–158, 1985.
6. Aaron DJ, Kriska AM, Dearwater SR, et al. The epidemiology of leisure physical activity in an adolescent population. *Med Sci Sports Exerc* 25:847–853, 1993.
7. Anonymous: Pondering how to squeeze fitness programs into schools' budgetary, time constraints. *JAMA* 616–617, 1992.

8. Stephens T: Secular trends in adult physical activity: Exercise boom or bust? *Res Q Exerc Sport* 58:94–105, 1987.
9. Jacobs DR Jr, Hahn LP, Folsom AR, et al: Time trends in leisure-time physical activity in the upper Midwest 1957–1987: University of Minnesota studies. *Epidemiology* 2:8–15, 1991.
10. Caspersen CJ, Pollard RA, Pratt SO: Scoring physical activity data with special consideration for elderly populations. In *Proceedings of the 21st National Meeting of the Public Health Conference on Records and Statistics: Data for An Aging Population, July 13–15, 1987*. D.H.H.S. Pub. No. (PHS) 88-1214, Hyattsville, Md.: U.S. Department of Health and Human Services, Public Health Service, Centers for Disease Control, National Center for Health Statistics, 1988, pp. 30–34.
11. Caspersen CJ, Merritt RK: Physical activity trends among 26 states, 1986–1990. *Med Sci Sports Exerc* 27:713–720, 1995.
12. Spencer G: *Projections of the Population of the United States, by Age, Sex, and Race: 1983–2080*. Washington, D.C.: U.S. Bureau of the Census, 1989.
13. Dishman RK, Sallis FJ, Orenstein DR: The determinants of physical activity and exercise. *Public Health Rep* 100:158–171, 1985.
14. Dishman RK: Increasing and maintaining physical activity and exercise. *Behav Ther* 22:345–378, 1991.
15. Hovell MF, Sallis JF, Hofstetter CR, et al: Identifying correlates of walking for exercise: An epidemiologic prerequisite for physical activity promotion. *Prev Med* 18:856–866, 1989.
16. Sallis JF, Haskell WL, Fortmann SP, et al: Predictors of adoption and maintenance of physical activity in a community sample. *Prev Med* 15:331–341, 1986.
17. Treiber FA, Baranowski T, Braden DS, et al: A descriptive epidemiology of leisure-time physical fitness rather than physical activity? *Am J Epidemiol* 125:601–610, 1987.
18. Kriska AM, Bayles JA, Cauley RE et al: A randomized exercise trial in older women: Increased activity over two years and the factors associated with compliance. *Med Sci Sports Exerc* 18:557–562, 1986.
19. Dishman RK: Exercise adherence research: Future direction. *Am J Health Promotion* 3:52–56, 1988.
20. Carmody TP, Senner JW, Manilow MR, et al: Physical exercise rehabilitation: Long-term dropout rate in cardiac patients. *J Behav Med* 3:163–168, 1980.
21. Dishman RK: Compliance/adherence in health-related exercise. *Health Psych* 1:237–267, 1982.
22. Dishman RK: Overview. In Dishman RK (ed): *Exercise Adherence*. Champaign, Ill, Human Kinetics, 1988, pp 1–9.
23. Prochaska JO, DiClemente CC. Stages and processes of self-change in smoking: Toward an integrative model of change. *J Consult Clin Psych* 51:390–395, 1983.
24. Prochaska JO, DiClemente CC: *The Transtheoretical Approach: Crossing the Traditional Boundaries of Therapy*. Homewood, Ill, Dow-Jones/Irwin, 1984.
25. Prochaska JO, DiClemente CC: Common processes of self-change in smoking, weight control, and psychological distress. In Shiffman S, Wills T (eds): *Coping and Substance Use*. New York, Academic Press, 1985, pp 345–363.
26. Prochaska JO, DiClemente CC: Toward a comprehensive model of change. In Miller WR, Heather N (eds): *Treating Addictive Behaviors: Processes of Change*. New York: Plenum Press, 1986, pp 3–27.
27. Prochaska JO, DiClemente CC: Stages of change in the modification of problem behaviors. In Hersen M, Eisler RM, Miller PM (eds): *Progress in behavior Modification*. Newbury Park, Calif, Sage, 1992, pp. 184–218.

28. Dubbert PM: Exercise in behavioral medicine. *J Consult Clin Psych* 60:613–618, 1992.
29. Sonstroem RJ: Psychological models. In Dishman RK (ed): *Exercise Adherence.* Champaign, Ill, Human Kinetics, 1988, pp. 125–154.
30. Velicer WF, DiClemente CC, Rossi JS, et al: Relapse situations and self-efficacy: An integrative model. *Addict Behav* 15:271–283, 1990.
31. D'Zurilla TJ: *Problem Solving Therapy: A Social Competence Approach to Clinical Intervention.* New York, Springer, 1986.
32. Nezu AM: Efficacy of a social problem-solving therapy approach for unipolar depression. *J Consult Clin Psych* 54:196–202, 1986.
33. Black DR, Scherba DS: Contracting to problem solve versus contracting to practice behavioral weight loss skills. *Behav Ther* 14:100–109, 1983.
34. Ewart CK: Social action theory for a public health psychology. *Am Psychol* 46:931–946, 1981.
35. Valente CM, Sobal J, Muncie HL et al: Health promotion: Physicians' beliefs, attitudes, and practices. *Am J Prev Med* 2:82–88, 1982.
36. Leon AS, Connett J: Physical activity and 10.5 year mortality in the Multiple Risk Factor Intervention Trial (MRFIT). *Int J Epidemiol* 20:690–697, 1991.
37. Lie H, Mundal R, Erikssen J: Coronary risk factors and incidence of coronary death in relation to physical fitness: Seven-year follow-up study of middle-aged and elderly men. *Eur Heart J* 6:147–156, 1985.
38. O'Connor GR, Buring JE, Yusuf S, et al: An overview of randomized trials of rehabilitation with exercise after myocardial infarction. *Circulation* 80:234–244, 1989.
39. Paffenbarger RS, Hyde RT, Wing AL, et al: A natural history of athleticism and cardiovascular health. *JAMA* 252:491–495, 1984.
40. Paffenberger RS, Hyde RT, Wing AL et al: The association of changes in physical-activity level and other lifestyle characteristics with mortality among men. *N Engl J Med* 328:538–545, 1993.
41. Peters RK, Cady LD, Bischoff DP, et al: Physical fitness and subsequent myocardial infarction in healthy workers. *JAMA* 249:3052–3056, 1983.
42. Powell KE, Thompson PD, Caspersen CJ, et al: Physical activity and the incidence of coronary heart disease. *Ann Rev Public Health* 8:253–287, 1987.
43. Sandvik L, Erikssen J, Thaulow E, et al: Physical fitness as a predictor of mortality among healthy, middle-aged Norwegian men. *N Engl J Med* 328:533–537, 1993.
44. Saltin B. Cardiovascular and pulmonary adaptation to physical activity. In Bouchard C, Shephard RJ, Stephens T, et al (eds): *Exercise, Fitness, and Health.* Champaign, Ill, Human Kinetics, 1988, pp 187–204.
45. Sutton JR, Farrell PA, Harber VJ: Hormonal adaptation to physical activity. In Bouchard C, Shephard RJ, Stephens T, et al (eds): *Exercise, Fitness, and Health.* Champaign, Ill, Human Kinetics, 1988, pp 217–258.
46. Bjorntorp P: Adipose tissue adaptation to exercise. In Bouchard C, Shephard RJ, Stephens T, et al (eds): *Exercise, Fitness, and Health.* Champaign, Ill, Human Kinetics, 1988, pp 315–324.
47. Blair SN, Kohl HW, Brill PA: Behavioral adaptation to physical activity. In Bouchard C, Shephard RJ, Stephens T, (eds): *Exercise, Fitness, and Health.* Champaign, Ill, Human Kinetics, 1988, pp 385–398.
48. Anonymous: Public health focus: Physical activity and the prevention of coronary heart disease. *MMWR* 42:669–672, 1993.
49. Arroll B, Beaglehole R: Does physical activity lower blood pressure: A critical review of the clinical trials. *J Clin Epidemiol* 45:439–447, 1992.

50. Seals DR, Hagberg JM: The effect of exercise training on human hypertension: A review. *Med Sci Sports Exerc* 16:207–215, 1984.
51. Hagberg JM: Exercise, fitness, and hypertension. In Bouchard C, Shephard RJ, Stephens T, et al (eds): *Exercise, Fitness, and Health.* Champaign, Ill, Human Kinetics, 1990, pp 455–462.
52. Paffenberger RS Jr, Wing Al, Hyde RT, et al: Physical activity and incidence of hypertension in college alumni. *Am J Epidemiol* 117:245–257, 1983.
53. Arroll B, Beaglehole R: Does physical activity lower blood pressure?: A critical review of the clinical trials. *J Clin Epidemiol* 45:439–447, 1992.
54. Blair SN, Goodyear NN, Gibbons LW, et al: Physical fitness an incidence of hypertension in healthy normotensive men and women. *JAMA* 252:487–490, 1984.
55. Bjorntorp PMD: Hypertension and exercise. *Hypertension.* 4(V pt 2):III56–III59, 1982.
56. Hagberg JM, Montain SJ, Martin WH, et al: Effect of exercise training on 60–69 year old persons with essential hypertension. *Am J Cardiol* 52:763–768, 1989.
57. Jennings GL, Deak G, Korner P, et al: What is the dose–response relationship between exercise training and blood pressure? *Ann Med* 23:313–318, 1991.
58. Haskell WL: The influence of exercise on the concentrations of triglyceride and cholesterol in human plasma. *Exerc Sport Sci Rev* 12:205–244, 1984.
59. Haskell WL: Exercise-induced changes in plasma lipids and lipoproteins. *Prev Med* 13:23–26, 1984.
60. Juneau M, Rogers F, DeSantos V, et al: Effectiveness of self-monitored, home-based moderate-intensity exercise training in middle-aged men and women. *Am J Cardiol* 60:66–70, 1987.
61. King AC, Haskell WL, Taylor CB et al: Group-versus home-based exercise training in healthy older men and women: A community-based clinical trial. *JAMA* 266:1525–1542, 1991.
62. Haskell WL, Taylor HL, Wood PD, et al: Strenuous physical activity, treadmill exercise test performance and plasma high-density lipoprotein cholesterol: The Lipid Research Clinics Program Prevalence Study. *Circulation* 62 (4P + 2):iv53–61, 1980.
63. King H, Kriska AM: Prevention of type II diabetes by physical training. Epidemiological considerations and study methods. *Diab Care* 15:1794–1799, 1992.
64. Eriksson KF, Lindgarde F: Prevention of type 2 (non-insulin-dependent) diabetes mellitus by diet and physical exercise. The 6-year Malmo feasibility study. *Diabetologia* 34:891–898, 1991.
65. Uusitupa M: Hypertension in diabetic patients—use of exercise in treatment. *Ann Med* 23:335–338, 1991.
66. Krotkiewski M, Bjorntorp P: Muscle tissue in obesity with different distribution of adipose tissue. Effects of physical training. *Int J Obes* 10:331–341, 1986.
67. Vansant G, Den Besten C, Weststrate J, et al: Body fat distribution and the prognosis for weight reduction: Preliminary observations. *In J Obes* 12:133–140, 1988.
68. Hjermann I: The metabolic cardiovascular syndrome: Syndrome X, Reaven's syndrome, insulin resistance syndrome, atherothrombogenic syndrome. *J Cardiovasc Pharm* 20(Suppl 8):S5–S10, 1992.
69. Klesges RC, Klesges LM, Haddock CK, et al: A longitudinal analysis of the impact of dietary intake and physical activity on weight change in adults. *Am J Clin Nutr* 55:818–822, 1992.
70. Folsom AR, Qamhieh HT, Flack JM, et al: Plasma fibrinogen levels and correlates in young adults. The Coronary Artery Risk Development in Young Adults (CARDIA) Study. *Am J Epidemiol* 138:1023–1036, 1993.

71. Neuhaus D, Gaehtgens P: Haemorrheology and long term exercise. *Sports Med* 18:10–21, 1994.
72. Williams RS, Logue EE, Lewis J, et al. Physical conditioning augments the fibrinolytic response to venous occlusion in healthy adults. *N Engl J Med* 302:987–991, 1980.
73. Lee I, Paffenbarger RS. Physical activity and its relation to cancer risk: A prospective study of college alumni. *Med Sci Sports Exerc* 26:831–837, 1994.
74. Berstein L, Henderson BE, Hanisch R, et al. Physical exercise and reduced risk of breast cancer in young women. *J Natl Cancer Inst* 86:1371–1372, 1994.
75. Plante T, Rodin J. Physical fitness and enhanced psychological health. *Curr Psychol* 9:3–24.
76. Shepard RJ, Rhind S, Shek PN: Exercise and the immune system. Natural killer cells, interleukins, and related responses. *Sports Med* 18:340–369, 1994.
77. Mittleman MA, Maclure M, Tofler GH, et al: Triggering of acute myocardial infarction by heavy physical exertion. Protection against triggering by regular exertion. Determinants of myocardial infarction onset study investigators. *N Engl J Med* 329:1677–1683, 1993.
78. Jones BH, Cowan DN, Knapik JJ: Exercise, training, and injuries. *Sports Med* 18:202–214, 1994.
79. Jones BH, Cowan DN, Tomlinson JP, et al: Epidemiology of injuries associated with physical training among young men in the army. *Med Sci Sports Exerc* 25:197–203, 1993.
80. Oldridge NB, Guyatt G, Jones N, et al: Effects on quality of life with comprehensive rehabilitation after cute myocardial infarction. *Am J Cardiol* 67:1084–1089, 1991.
81. Pilote L, Thomas RJ, Dennis C, et al: Return to work after uncomplicated myocardial infarction: A trial of practice guidelines in the community. *Ann Intern Med* 117:383–389, 1992.
82. Housley E, Leng GC, Donnan PT, et al: Physical activity and risk of peripheral arterial disease in the general population: Edinburgh Artery Study. *J Epidemiol Community Health* 47(6):475–480, 1993.
83. Sidoti SP: Exercise and peripheral vascular disease. *Clin Podiatr Med Surg* 9:173–184, 1992.
84. Haskell WL: The efficacy and safety of exercise programs in cardiac rehabilitation. *Med Sci Sports Exerc* 26:815–823, 1994.
85. Van Camp SP, Peterson PA: Cardiovascular complications of outpatient cardiac rehabilitation programs. *JAMA* 256:1160–1163, 1986.
86. Kottke TE, Brekke ML, Solberg LI: Making "time" for preventative services. *Mayo Clin Proc* 68:785–791, 1993.
87. Wells KB, Ware JE, Lewis CE: Physicians' practices in counseling patients about health habits. *Med Care* 22:240–246, 1984.
88. Mullen P, Tabak GR: Patterns of counseling techniques used by family practice physicians for smoking, weight, exercise, and stress. *Med Care* 27:694–704, 1989.
89. National Center for Health Statistics, U.S. Department of Health and Human Services: *Physician Visits: Volume and Interval Since Last Visit, United States, 1980.* DHHS Pub. No. (PHS) 83-1572.
90. Philips BU Jr, Longoria JM, Calhoun KH, et al: Behavioral prescription writing in smoking cessation counseling: A new use for a familiar tool. *South Med J* 82:946–953, 1989.
91. Logsdon DN, Lazaro CM, Meier RV: The feasibility of behavior risk reduction in primary medical care. *Am J Prev Med* 5:249–256, 1989.
92. DeBusk RF, Miller NH, Superko HR, et al: A case management system for coronary risk factor modification following acute myocardial infarction. *Ann Intern Med* 120:721–729, 1994.

◆ CHAPTER TWO ◆

ADAPTATIONS TO EXERCISE: IMPLICATIONS FOR PATIENTS WITH CARDIOVASCULAR DISORDERS

Carl Foster, Ph.D

INTRODUCTION

The Greek legend of the young farmer who lifted a calf daily as the calf grew into a bull, thus becoming a legendary strongman, defines the primary operating expectation about exercise training: do something that is physically challenging with some degree of regularity, and that which was difficult becomes routine. The ability to adapt to exercise is also important for patients with cardiovascular disease. By the time of the American Revolution, Herberden[1] had published the observation that one of his patients with heart disease (probably exertional angina pectoris) was nearly cured after a daily half hour of sawing wood. In the two decades following the publication of *Aerobics*[2] by Dr Ken Cooper, following the pioneering work of Drs. Bruno Balke, Myrvin Ellestad, Herman Hellerstein, Albert Kattus, and Paul Dudley White, there was much interest in the therapeutic possibilities of exercise for the prevention and treatment of cardiovascular disease. This led to a belief on the part of some that if one were to exercise enough (e.g., run a marathon), one would be virtually immune from cardiovascular disease.[3] Even though these claims were ultimately refuted,[4] there remains a widespread belief that more, and more vigorous, exercise is better, On the other hand, professional societies as important as the American College of Sports Medicine and the Centers for Disease Control have recently published a position stand suggesting that the exercise training load necessary to derive the health benefits of exercise may be much less than had been thought during the 1970s and 1980s.[5] What are physicians to tell their patients? What can realistically be expected from participation in systematic exercise training?

CASE EXAMPLE

Patient History and Examination

A 58-year-old woman who suffered an uncomplicated myocardial infarction 2 weeks ago presents in your office with questions about the physical activities she can safely perform. She has two chronic conditions which are well controlled by diet and drugs: hypertension, for which she takes atenolol and enalapril, and hypercholesterolemia, for which she takes simvistatin. She has been without angina since her discharge from the hospital 1 week ago. She walks slowly for 10 min each day, covering approximately two blocks at a time.

The patient undergoes an exercise treadmill test in your office and is able to achieve a maximal exercise capacity approximately equivalent to 9 METS. At peak exercise she develops chest discomfort, along with 1 mm of ST depression in the lateral ECG leads. The chest discomfort resolves during the first minute of recovery, and the ischemic ECG changes resolve by 3 min into recovery.

Comments/Questions

What physiologic adaptations can this patient expect to experience during her participation in an exercise program? Will her fitness improve or will it be limited by her angina? Is it likely that an exercise program will improve her left ventricular structure or function? Will her myocardial perfusion improve?

CHANGES IN EXERCISE CAPACITY

With very few exceptions, the one sure thing that can be said about exercise training is that exercise capacity will improve. This can most easily be noted by increases in exercise duration during standard clinical exercise tests. However, because exercise tests are primarily composed of low-intensity submaximal stages, the magnitude of increase in exercise duration (usually no more than 2 min on a standard Bruce treadmill protocol) can underestimate the change in exercise capacity that is apparent to the patient.

Physiologists often use maximal pulmonary oxygen uptake (VO_2max) as the definitive index of adaptation to exercise training. Indeed, early consensus work done with the World Health Organization virtually defined VO_2max as equivalent to the concept of endurance and, in so doing, provided the impetus for the many experimental exercise training studies in the 1970s and 1980s. VO_2max represents the physiologic integration of maximal cardiac output and arteriovenous oxygen difference. Since variations in the maximal arteriovenous oxygen difference between individuals are comparatively small, VO_2max represents a fairly good index of maximal cardiac output.[6] In both healthy sedentary adults and clinically stable patients with cardiovascular disease, VO_2max may be expected to increase 15–30% with 6 months to 1 year of regular exercise training (Figure 2-1). Beyond this, there is comparatively little further increase in VO_2max with continued training.

VO_2max is most representative of the intensity of exercise that can be sustained for 3–7 min. It probably does not represent an exercise intensity voluntarily undertaken by many individuals outside the confines of the athletic arena or exercise laboratory. Most patients, rather, have a clearer sense of the exercise capacity that is sustainable for 30–60 min of hard work. During the last decade, attempts to define sustainable exercise tolerance have made great strides. Observations, primarily in Europe, of the pattern of blood lactate accumulation during exercise and, primarily in the United States, of the pattern of pulmonary ventilation during exercise have suggested a strategy for quantifying sustainable exercise tolerance.[7] Sustainable

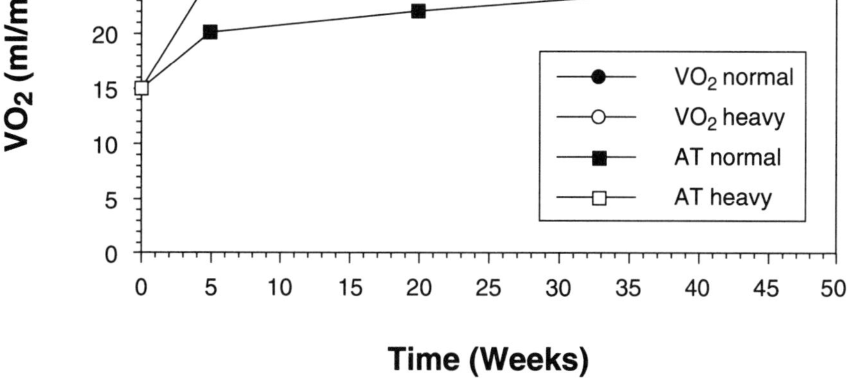

FIGURE 2-1. Changes in VO_2max and sustainable exercise tolerance (AT) during normal training (three to four times weekly at 75% HRmax)(closed symbols) and during heavy training (five to seven times weekly at 85% HRmax)(open symbols) in clinically stable patients with an initial VO_2max of 30 ml/min/kg and a sustainable exercise tolerance of 50% VO_2max. Note both the faster early increase in exercise capacity and the more extensive total increase with heavier training.

exercise tolerance typically averages 50–70% of VO_2max. The more highly trained the individual, the higher the %VO_2max represented by the sustainable exercise tolerance. Depending on the strategy for defining sustainable exercise tolerance, a wide variety of terms are used, including *anaerobic threshold, ventilatory threshold, lactate threshold, onset of blood lactate accumulation,* and *individual anaerobic threshold.* Sustainable exercise tolerance may continue to improve for up to 2–3 years with continued exercise, with a ultimate increase of up to 100% of the pre-training value (Figure 2-1).

Most of the improved exercise tolerance with exercise training occurs comparatively rapidly, that is, within a few months.[8] However, as noted above, sustainable exercise capacity can continue to improve for some period of time. There is something of a dose–response character to both the magnitude and time course of improved exercise tolerance with training. With three to four 30- to 60-min exercise sessions per week, ~90% of the potential improvement in VO_2max and ~50% of the potential improvement in sustainable exercise tolerance may be expected to occur within 6 months. Exercise training intensity is more important than frequency or duration for changes in VO_2max and sustainable exercise tolerance. Recent studies by Franklin et al.[9,10] have demonstrated that patients completing a maximal exercise test (~10 min duration) three times weekly for 6 weeks increased their VO_2max and ventilatory threshold significantly more than patient engaged in conventional exercise training at 70–85% maximal heart rate for 30 min. Although the sustainable exercise tolerance may ultimately improve nearly 100% over pretraining values, this usually requires almost daily exercise for an hour or more, including some fairly high intensity sessions. Given that few patients are likely to be willing to effectively become competitive athletes, a more realistic expectation is a 50–60% increase in sustainable exercise tolerance after 1 to 2 years of regular exercise training.

IMPROVED SYMPTOMS AND QUALITY OF LIFE

Regardless of the change in objectively measured exercise capacity (whether VO_2-max or sustainable exercise capacity), most patients note a significant reduction in symptoms (angina pectoris, dyspnea, or claudication, for example) following exercise training. As alluded to earlier, this reduction in symptoms was noted over two centuries ago.[1] The ability of exercise training to minimize symptoms was also important in the rediscovery of the value of structured exercise for patients with cardiovascular disease following World War II. Much of the reduction in symptoms following exercise training may be attributed to the reduced heart rate and blood pressure required for standard tasks following exercise training. Many studies suggest a reduction in heart rate during standard exercise bouts of about 10–20 beats per minute at the workload associated with the sustainable exercise capacity before training. This is comparable to the effect achieved by consuming 20–40 mg daily of propranolol and led to the early suggestion that exercise training was nature's own beta blocker.[11]

Recent studies have suggested that even patients with chronic congestive heart failure may benefit symptomatically from exercise training, even though the left ventricular ejection fraction does not change systematically and even though these patients still suffer periodic episodes of congestive heart failure and a comparatively high mortality rate.[12,13] These studies also suggest that increases in cardiac output are associated with the early increase in VO_2max and exercise capacity and that changes in lactate metabolism are responsible for the continuing change in exercise capacity with more long-term training. The skeletal muscles' adaptations to exercise may allow minimization of the cardiac output required to do defined submaximal tasks and a reduction of the high systemic vascular resistance in these patients.

In addition, patients commonly report that they feel better and can do more things that are meaningful to them following exercise training. This observation has been lumped under the rubic of "quality of life." For many years, quality of life was considered something of a soft endpoint and not clinically significant. However, in recent years, well-validated scales for measuring quality of life have emerged.[14–16] The best contemporary data suggest that quality of life improves independently of changes in objective exercise capacity.[7] In particular, the recovery of an acceptable quality of life following an acute clinical episode is much more rapid than objective exercise capacity measured by cycle ergometry. Interpretation of quality of life is still hampered by the partially overlapping nature of the different scales used and by the lack of data to define the normal range of variation. In fairly typical patients participating in an outpatient rehabilitation program, substantial changes in quality of life are possible within 12 weeks (Figure 2-2).

Patients also tend to report greater self-efficacy, or confidence in their ability to engage in various activities, following participation in exercise-based rehabilitation programs.[7] Early studies on the concept of self-efficacy demonstrated that what patients believe they are able to do defines their subsequent actions more than does their objective exercise tolerance.[17] Early studies also demonstrated that self-efficacy was specific to the type of activity undertaken, implying that practice with an activity in a supportive atmosphere may be as important to increasing self-efficacy as actual physiologic adaptations.[18] Like quality of life, self-efficacy improves more rapidly than objective exercise tolerance.[7]

IMPROVED RISK FACTORS

The multifactorial nature of the development and progression of cardiovascular disease is well documented. It is probably fair to say that the direct effect of exercise training on conventional risk factors is modest. Although there is a known tendency for HDL cholesterol to increase, for blood pressure to decrease (at least transiently[19]), and for glucose tolerance to improve slightly, the direct effect of exercise training on conventional risk factors is not large.

In light of our emerging understanding of the importance of patients taking responsibility for their treatment and the critical importance of mind–body interactions in disease states, the indirect effects of exercise training may be of great importance. First, exercise training is something that patients do for themselves.

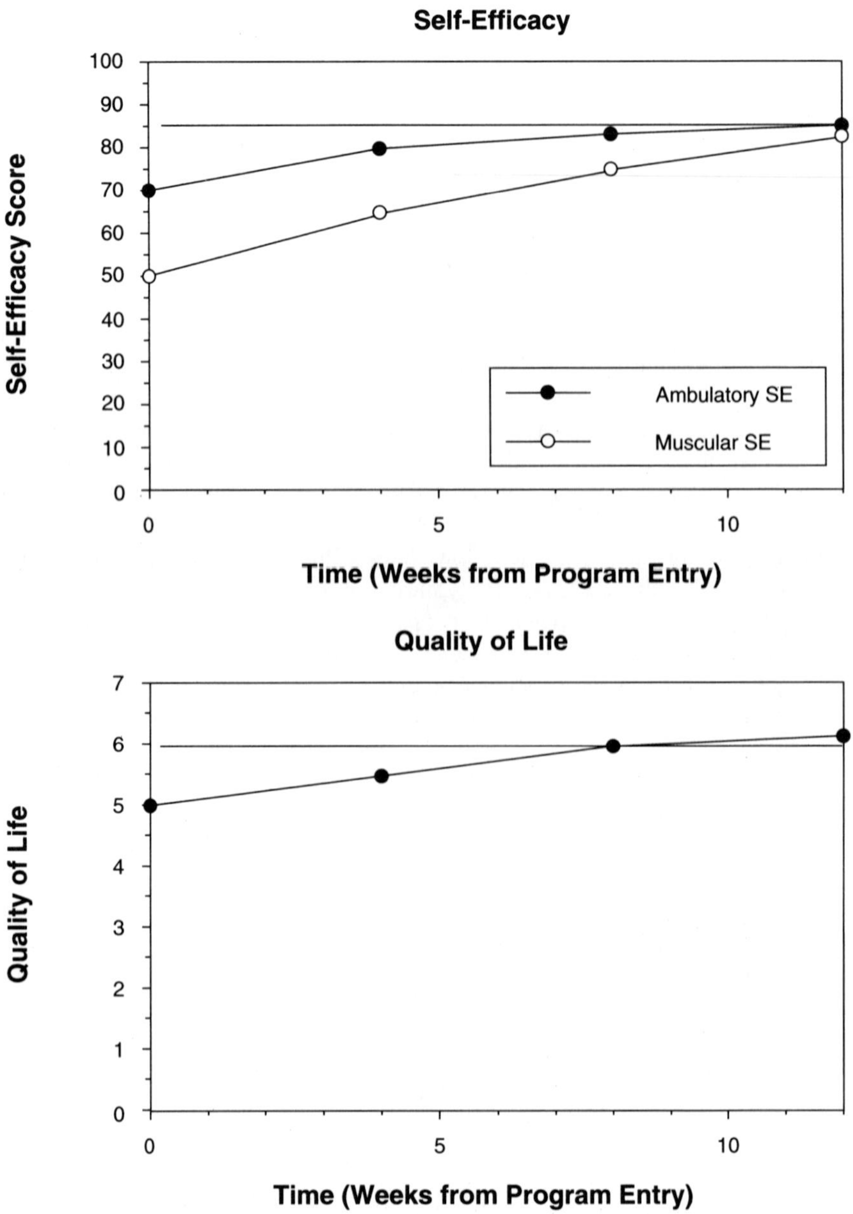

FIGURE 2-2. Temporal pattern of changes in the self-efficacy score and quality of life score during a conventional rehabilitation program. Although there is no established normal value for either self-efficacy or quality of life, we have indicated 85% of the possible range of variation as a nominal normal value. (Adapted from Ref. 8)

It is not a procedure that is done to them, and it is not a drug that is prescribed for them. With exercise training, patients largely direct and carry out their own therapy. Exercise advice from a health care professional also has the advantage of being positive. Given that people are less inclined to listen to negative advice (don't smoke, for example), however well intended, there is much to be said for positive advice.

Although contemporary studies do not fully support the regression hypothesis,[20] there is good evidence that many of the adaptations resulting form exercise training can act to stabilize atherosclerotic lesions[21] and enhance coronary vasodilatory capacity,[22] resulting in a reduced risk of clinical episodes, a prediction supported by clinical observations.[23] The easily observable improvement in exercise capacity consequent to systematic training can, additionally, foster hope that patients can recover from their disease with minimal disruption in their lifestyle. This may, in turn, foster greater satisfaction with the treatment process. In the mid-1990s, the importance of patient satisfaction with the outcome of therapy can hardly be overstated.

In addition to strictly physiologic adaptations, closely related psychological adaptations can occur with exercise training. When properly done, exercise can represent "time out" from work, from family responsibilities, from the phone, and from the fax machine. The effect of exercise on anxiety is similar, in fact, to that of periods of quiet time or even meditation.[24] Given the potential importance of psychophysiologic factors for vascular tone and the presentation of cardiovascular symptoms,[25–27] strategies like exercise designed to remove the patient from stressful environments are of potentially great importance.

There is something of a paradox in that the focus and intensity of exercise necessary to elicit maximal physiologic adaptations[9,10] are the opposite of the mild, rhythmic, noncompetitive exercise designed to promote psychophysiologic adaptations.[28] In this regard, it is worth noting that the single death in the Lifestyle Trial reported by Ornish et al. occurred in a rather fit patient who maintained a very competitive attitude toward his extensive exercise training and who died shortly after "beating the computer" on a electronic rowing machine.[29] Further, recent studies demonstrate that the risk of exercise-induced myocardial infarction in previously sedentary individuals is primarily related to unusual exercise intensity.[30,31] Thus, although patients can participate in highly strenuous activities including marathon running,[32] mountain hiking,[33] cross-country skiing,[34] and swimming,[35] and may even garner greater physiologic benefits from such activities,[36] there is a demonstrable risk from a psychophysiologic perspective.

CHANGES IN VENTRICULAR STRUCTURE

There is a fairly extensive literature detailing the changes in left ventricular structure consequent to exercise training. Much of the early literature focused on differences in ventricular structure in athletic individuals trained for different sports. These data led to the early suggestion that aerobic training resulted in an increase in left ventricular chamber size without a large change in wall thickness, whereas resistance training led to an increase in wall thickness with no change in left ventricular chamber size. More contemporary longitudinal studies have suggested that aerobic training leads to a more or less proportional increase in left ventricular dimensions.[37] In many early clinical studies, there was remarkably little evidence of changes in left ventricular dimensions following participation in rehabilitation programs. Only studies which included comparatively severe exercise training, similar to that undertaken by younger and healthier individuals, reported evidence of increases in left ventricular size. Thus, just as acquiring large skeletal muscles requires fairly intense training, changes in left ventricular structure consequent to exercise training may only be expected following fairly severe exercise training programs.

Some concern was generated a few years ago by reports that exercise training soon after anterior myocardial infarction was associated with extension of the infarct-related scar.[38] This raised the possibility that rehabilitation programs should be delayed until the scar resulting from the myocardial infarction had time to fully develop. However, recent studies[39] using carefully matched patients who either exercised three times weekly from week 8 to week 20 after myocardial infarction demonstrated no increase in the percentage of abnormal wall motion or endocardial surface area–body surface area index. Thus it would seem that the risk of adverse left ventricular remodeling with exercise training is low. Likewise, although there are only a few case reports of left ventricular rupture with exercise following acute myocardial infarction, the general recommendation to delay severe exercise for approximately 6 weeks following infarction is probably reasonable, commonsense advice.

CHANGES IN VENTRICULAR FUNCTION

A variety of studies have examined changes in cardiac output in response to training in patients with cardiovascular disease. These studies are well represented by the recent report of Szmedra et al., which found minimal changes in cardiac output despite increases in exercise tolerance and VO_2max in patients with either normal or depressed left ventricular ejection fractions.[40] However, this study used CO_2 rebreathing to measure cardiac output during submaximal exercise. No direct measures of peak cardiac output were made. Recent studies using direct Fick measures of cardiac output during exercise training in patients with very low left ventricular ejection fractions (<40%) demonstrated that the main contributor to an increase in power output during the first month of training was increased cardiac output.[10] Thereafter, although there was a continued increase in exercise capacity, further changes in cardiac output were minimal.

Well-trained, healthy individuals usually have somewhat higher values for peak exercise left ventricular ejection fraction than do sedentary individuals.[41] In healthy individuals, there is usually no systematic change in left ventricular ejection fraction following exercise training.[42] Further, there are minimal changes in peak exercise left ventricular ejection fraction following training in patients with stable ischemia[43,44] or following myocardial revascularization surgery.[45] Results from our earlier study[45] suggest that the increase in exercise capacity with exercise training following myocardial revascularization surgery may be accounted for by increases in cardiac output resulting from increases in peak heart rate and stroke volume. Changes in stroke volume can easily be accounted for by small increases in exercise end-diastolic volume. Although the left ventricular ejection fraction does not change with training, there is apparently no reduction in the ability to increase VO_2max with training in patients with low values for left ventricular ejection fraction.[40]

CHANGES IN MYOCARDIAL PERFUSION

Early studies demonstrated that the product of heart rate and systolic blood pressure (the rate pressure product, a measure of myocardial oxygen demand) at peak exercise was very stable in patients with coronary heart disease, even following exercise training. This led to the belief that myocardial perfusion was not responsive to training. However, beginning in the early 1980s, a series of studies with more aggressive interventions demonstrated an increased rate–pressure product,[46–48] myocardial perfusion by thallium scintigraphy,[43,44,49,10] and quantitative angiography.[29,51–53] These results may be related to regression of coronary lesions, although the absolute changes in lesion size are usually quite small.[21] Alternatively, systematic exercise may increase the vasodilatory reserve of the coronary arteries.[22,53–55] Recent cross-sectional data using intracoronary artery ultrasound have demonstrated a relationship between the potential increase in coronary artery blood flow and VO_2max.[56] If these data hold true for longitudinal changes in VO_2max, the first true demonstration of exercise training–induced changes in coronary blood flow will have been made.

POTENTIAL RISKS OF EXERCISE

Exercise is a very safe activity, as noted in Chapter 1. Statistics concerning the risks of exercise training in both healthy individuals and patients with coronary artery disease suggest that the risk of untoward events is on the order of 0.1–0.3 per 10,000 hours of training.[57–59] Assuming 2.5 hr per week per individual,[5] this represents one untoward event per year per 1000 patients. Given that most witnessed events can be managed fairly successfully, the likelihood of a serious untoward event seems quite small. Recent data suggest that in previously sedentary individuals, high-intensity exercise may be associated with the development of acute myocardial infarction.[30,31] This is consistent with the demonstration that the risk of untoward events in rehabilitation programs is associated with definable risk factors, including relatively good exercise tolerance, demonstrable ischemia during exercise testing, and frequent violation of the target heart rate during training.[60] Taken together, these results suggest that exercise during ischemia may be undesirable. Some studies have suggested that exertional ischemia may result in myocardial "stunning."[61,62] Recent studies in our laboratory have demonstrated that left ventricular function is fundamentally stable during 30 min of exercise training in patients with exertional ischemia.[63] These results are consistent with the concept of "walk-through angina" or "second-effort angina"[64,65] and imply that there is a slow autoregulation of myocardial blood flow during prolonged exercise. From this, it may be inferred that the primary risk of high-intensity exercise in patients with ischemia is related to acute plaque rupture or to arrhythmias. Accordingly, high-intensity exercise (or exercise above the ischemic threshold) should probably be undertaken only in the presence of adequate monitoring and resuscitative capability.

SUMMARY

1. Under most circumstances, exercise promotes beneficial physiologic and psychological adaptations for patients with cardiovascular disease. Exercise training certainly provokes favorable adaptations in both objective and subjective markers of exercise capacity and contributes to an improved quality of life.
2. At higher exercise training loads, there may be improvements in risk factors, myocardial perfusion, and ventricular function related to exercise training.
3. Exercise may serve as both "time out" from the stressors of everyday life and a positive focus for necessary lifestyle changes.
4. Many of the physiologic adaptations associated with exercise training seem to be related to higher exercise training intensities. However, higher exercise intensities are also associated with most of the comparatively rare complications observed during exercise training. Accordingly, it is probably desirable to start exercise training at relatively low intensities and to increase intensity gradually as tolerated.

REFERENCES

1. Heberden W: Commentaries on the history and cure of disease. In Williams FA, Keys TW (eds): *Classics in Cardiology.* New York, Dover, 1961.
2. Cooper KH: *Aerobics*. New York, Bantam Books, 1968.
3. Bassler TJ: Marathon vs distance running. *N Engl J Med* 294:114–118, 1976.
4. Handler JB, Asay RW, Warren SE: Symptomatic coronary artery disease in a marathon runner. *JAMA* 248:717–719, 1982.
5. Pate RR, Pratt M, Blair SN: Physical activity and public health: A recommendation from the Centers for Disease Control and Prevention and the American College of Sports Medicine. *JAMA* 273:402–407, 1995.
6. Weber KT, Janicki JS: *Cardiopulmonary Exercise Testing*. Philadelphia, WB Saunders, 1986.
7. Foster C, Schrager M, Snyder AC: Blood lactate and respiratory methods of evaluating the capacity for sustained exercise. In Maud PJ, Foster C (eds), *Physiological Assessment of Human Fitness.* Champaign, Ill, Human Kinetics, 1995, pp 57–72.
8. Foster C, Oldridge NB, Dion W, et al: Time course of recovery during cardiac rehabilitation. *J Cardiopulm Rehab* 15:209–215, 1995.
9. Franklin BA, Crause I, Bonzheim K, et al: Repeated maximal exercise testing—A stimulus for physical conditioning? *Circulation* 72:I-669, 1992.
10. Franklin BA, Crause I, Bonzheim K, et al: Ventilatory threshold alterations caused by repeated maximal exercise testing in sedentary men. *JACC* 21:431A, 1993.

11. Pollock ML, Wilmore JH: *Exercise in Health and Disease*, ed 2. Philadelphia, WB Saunders, 1990.
12. Dubach P, Meyers J, Dziekan G, et al: Central hemodynamics and gas exchange adaptations to training in chronic heart failure. *JACC* 25:21A, 1995.
13. Sullivan MJ, Higgenbotham MB, Cobb FR, et al: Exercise training in patients with severe left ventricular dysfunction: Hemodynamic and metabolic effects. *Circulation* 70:69–75, 1984.
14. Oldridge N, Guyatt G, Jones N: Effects on quality of life with comprehensive rehabilitation after acute myocardial infarction. *Am J Cardiol* 67:1084–1089, 1991.
15. Rector TS, Cohn JN: Assessment of patient outcome with the Minnesota Living With Heart Failure Questionnaire: Reliability and validity during a randomized, double blind, placebo controlled trial of pimobendan. *Am Heart J* 124:1017–1025, 1992.
16. Spertus JA, Winder JA, Dewhurst TA: Monitoring the quality of life in patients with coronary artery disease. *Am J Cardiol* 74:1240–1244, 1994.
17. Ewart CK, Taylor DB, Reese LB, et al: Effects of early postmyocardial infarction exercise training on self perceptions and subsequent physical activity. *Am J Cardiol* 51:1076–1080, 1983.
18. Taylor CB, Bandura A, Ewart CK, et al: Exercise testing to enhance wives' confidence in their husbands' cardiac capability soon after clinically uncomplicated myocardial infarction. *Am J Cardiol* 55:635–638, 1985.
19. Marceau M, Kouame N, Lacourciere Y, et al: Effects of different training intensities on 24 hour blood pressure in hypertensive subjects. *Circulation* 88:2803–2811, 1993.
20. Foster C, Schrager M, Cohen J: The value of cardiac rehabilitation: secondary prevention. In Pollack ML, Schmidt DG (eds): *Heart Disease and Rehabilitation*, ed 3. Champaign, Ill, Human Kinetics, 1994, pp 177–183.
21. Brown BG, Ahao XQ, Sacco DE: Lipid lowering and plaque regression: New insights into prevention of plaque disruption and clinical events in coronary disease. *Circulation* 87:1783–1791, 1993.
22. Haskell WL, Sims, C, Myll J: Coronary artery size and dilating capacity in ultradistance runners. *Circulation* 87:1076–1082, 1993.
23. Oldridge NB, Guyatt GH, Fischer MS: Cardiac rehabilitation after myocardial infarction: Combined experience of randomized clinical trials. *JAMA* 260:945–950, 1988.
24. Bahrke MS, Morgan WP: Anxiety reduction following exercise and meditation. *Cogn Ther Res* 2:323–334, 1978.
25. Rozanski A, Bairey CN, Krantz DS, et al: Mental stress and the induction of silent myocardial ischemia in patients with coronary artery disease. *N Engl J Med* 318:1005–1012, 1988.
26. Verrier RL, Hagestad EL, Lown B: Delayed myocardial ischemia induced by anger. *Circulation* 75:249–254, 1987.
27. Lacy CR, Contrada RJ, Robbins ML, et al: Coronary vasoconstriction induced by mental stress (simulated public speaking). *Am J Cardiol* 75:503–505, 1995.
28. Pearsall PK: The fifth factor in fitness: The connection between psychoneuroimmunology, cardiovascular and pulmonary health. *Proc AACVPR*, 1994.
29. Ornish D, Brown SE, Scherwitz LW: Can lifestyle changes reverse coronary heart disease? *Lancet* 336:129–133, 1990.
30. Mittleman MA, Maclure M, Tofler GH: Triggering of acute myocardial infarction by heavy physical exertion: Protection against triggering by regular exertion. *N Engl J Med* 329:1677–1683, 1993.
31. Willich SN, Lewis M, Lowel H, et al: Physical exertion as a trigger of acute myocardial infarction. *N Engl J Med* 329:1684–1690, 1993.

32. Kavanaugh T, Shephard RJ, Doney H, et al: Intensive exercise in coronary rehabilitation. *Med Sci Sports* 5:34–39, 1973.
33. Lehmann M, Durr H, Huonker M: Mountain hiking with CHD patients: Results of an experimental study. *Int J Sports Med* 14:173A, 1993.
34. Lehmann M, Huber G, Gastmann U: Heart rates, cardiac arrhythmia, lactate levels and catecholamine excretions in CHD patients during cross country skiing. *Int J Sports Med* 11:379–382, 1990.
35. Lehmann M. Samek L: Recreational swimming in CHD patients and healthy control subjects in relation to left heart function. *Clin Cardiol* 13:547–554, 1990.
36. Chandrashekhar Y, Anand IS: Exercise as a coronary protective factor. *Am Heart J* 122:1723–1739, 1991.
37. Foster C: Exercise training following cardiovascular surgery. *Exerc Sport Sci Rev* 14:303–324, 1986.
38. Judgutt BI, Michorowski BL, Cappagoda CT: Exercise training after anterior Q-wave myocardial infarction: Importance of regional let ventricular function and topography. *JACC* 12:363–372, 1988.
39. Cannistra LB, Davidoff R, Picard MH, et al: Does moderate to high intensity exercise affect left ventricular remodeling in cardiac rehabilitation patients after myocardial infarction? *JACC* 25:237A, 1995.
40. Szmedra L, Bacharach DW, Buckenmeyer PJ: Response of patients with coronary artery disease stratified by ejection fraction following short term training. *Int J Cardiol* 46:209–222, 1994.
41. Anholm JD, Foster C, Carpenter J, et al: Effect of habitual exercise on left ventricular response to exercise. *J Appl Physiol* 52:1648–1651, 1982.
42. Rerych SK, Scholtz PM, Sabiston DC, et al: Effect of exercise training on left ventricular function in normal subjects: A longitudinal study by radionuclide angiography. *Am J Cardiol* 45:244–250, 1980.
43. Verani MS, Hartund GH, Hoepful-Harris J: Effects of exercise training on left ventricular performance and myocardial perfusion in patients with coronary artery disease. *Am J Cardiol* 47:797–803, 1981.
44. Tubau J, Witzum K, Froelicher VF: Noninvasive assessment of changes in myocardial perfusion and ventricular performance following exercise training. *Am Heart J* 104:238–248, 1982.
45. Foster C, Pollock ML, Anholm JD: Work capacity and left ventricular function during rehabilitation after myocardial revascularization surgery. *Circulation* 69:748–755, 1984.
46. Ehsani AA, Heath GW, Hagberg JM: Effects of 12 months of intense exercise training on ischemic ST-segment depression in patients with coronary artery disease. *Circulation* 6:1116–1124, 1981.
47. Raffo JA, Luksic IY, Kappagoda CT: Effects of physical training on myocardial ischemia in patients with coronary artery disease. *Br Heart J* 43:262–269, 1980.
48. Laslett LJ, Paumer L, Amsterdam EA: Increase in myocardial oxygen consumption indexes by exercise training at onset of ischemia in patients with coronary artery disease. *Circulation* 71:958–962, 1985.
49. Froelicher VF, Jensen D, Genter R: A randomized trial of exercise training in patients with coronary heart disease. *JAMA* 252:1291–1297, 1984.
50. Schuler G, Schillert G, Wirth A: Low fat diet and regular supervised physical exercise in patients with symptomatic coronary artery disease: Reduction of stress induced myocardial ischemia. *Circulation* 77:172–181, 1988.
51. Gould KL, Ornish D, Kirkeeide D: Improved stenosis geometry by quantitative coronary arteriography after vigorous risk factor modification. *Am J Cardiol* 69:845–853, 1992.

52. Arntzenius AC, Kromhout D, Barth JD: Diet, lipoproteins and the progression of coronary atherosclerosis: The Liden intervention trial. *N Engl J Med* 312:805–811, 1985.
53. Haskell WL, Alderman EL, Fair JM: Effects of intensive multiple risk factor reduction on coronary atherosclerosis and clinical cardiac events in men and women with coronary artery disease: The Stanford Coronary Risk Intervention Project. *Circulation* 89:975–990, 1994.
54. Treasure CB, Klein JL, Weintraub WS, et al: Beneficial effects of cholesterol lowering therapy on the coronary endothelium in patients with coronary artery disease. *N Engl J Med* 332:481–487, 1995.
55. Anderson TJ, Meredith IT, Yeung AC, et al: The effect of cholesterol lowering and antioxidant therapy on endothelium dependent coronary vasomotion. *N Engl J Med* 332:488–493, 1995.
56. Joye JD, Flores AR, Orie JE, et al: Exercise capacity and coronary flow reserve in patients with intermediate coronary stenoses. *JACC* 25:259A, 1995.
57. Thompson PD, Funk EJ, Carleton RA, et al: Incidence of death during jogging in Rhode Island from 1975–1980. *JAMA* 247:2535–2538, 1982.
58. Haskell WL: Cardiovascular complications during exercise training of cardiac patients. *Circulation* 57:920–924, 1978.
59. Van Camp SP, Peterson RA: Cardiovascular complications of outpatient cardiac rehabilitation programs. *JAMA* 256:1160–1163, 1986.
60. Hossack K, Hartwig R: Cardiac arrest associated with supervised cardiac rehabilitation. *J Cardiopulm Rehabil* 2:402–408, 1982.
61. Kloner RA, Allen J, Cox TA: Stunned left ventricular myocardium after exercise treadmill testing in coronary artery disease. *Am J Cardiol* 68:329–334, 1991.
62. Masani N, Avery P, Jones R, et al: Prolonged myocardial dysfunction after exercise induced ischemia-myocardial stunning or delayed reperfusion. *JACC* 25:252A, 1995.
63. Foster C, Gal RA, Murphy P, et al: Ventricular function during exercise testing and training. *JACC* 25:260A, 1995.
64. McAlpin RN, Kattus AA: Adaptation to exercise in angina pectoris: The electrocardiogram during treadmill walking and coronary angiographic findings. *Circulation* 33:183–201, 1966.
65. Joy M, Cairns AW, Springings D: Observations on the warmup phenomenon in angina pectoris. *Br Heart J* 58:116–121, 1987.

♦ CHAPTER THREE ♦

BASIC PRINCIPLES OF PHYSICAL ACTIVITY COUNSELING: PROJECT PACE

Kevin Patrick, M.D., M.S.
Karen J. Calfas, Ph.D.
James F.Sallis, Ph.D.
Barbara Long, M.D.

INTRODUCTION

Clinicians have a unique and important role to play in counseling their patients to become physically active. This chapter aims to give readers the knowledge and tools for a systematic approach to physical activity counseling. It is based on over 4 years of development work by a team of primary care physicians, psychologists, behavioral and educational researchers, and medical office support staff. The goal for Project PACE—Physician-based Assessment and Counseling for Exercise—was a simple one: to develop a physical activity counseling strategy that was quick and easy to use, efficacious, and highly acceptable to patients and providers. The development of PACE was supported by the U.S. Public Health Service's Centers for Disease Control (CDC) to address one of the national health objectives for the Year 2000: to increase to at least 50% the percentage of primary care providers who appropriately assess and counsel their patients about physical activity.[1]

The primary focus of the PACE approach to physical activity counseling has been to improve the health habits of *apparently healthy adults*, i.e., patients without signs or symptoms of cardiovascular disease. Those patients who already carry the diagnosis of cardiovascular disease or who have overt signs or symptoms should (as readers will see in this and other chapters) be thoroughly evaluated before embarking on any physical activity program. However, the principles of the PACE approach—systematic screening, matching message to need, guided follow-up, and the value of clinician effort—are useful for all patients and, once learned, are generalizable to many health concerns.

The role of increased physical activity in reducing the risk of cardiovascular disease and other chronic diseases is addressed in Chapters 1 and 2. The fact that over 50% of Americans do not engage in physical activity at a level high enough to gain significant health benefits[2] suggests the need for strategies to increase their physical activity levels. For a number of reasons, strategies aimed at improving clinicians' abilities in this area show great promise.[3] Most Americans indicate that their primary source of health information is their personal physician.[4] More than 75% see a physician at least once yearly.[5] Even though physicians have the opportunity to address physical activity, most do not, and when they do, the discussion is of limited duration.[6] Physicians counsel less often about physical activity than about other important health behaviors.[7] A number of factors limit clinician participation in physical activity counseling:

1. *Lack of training, skill, and perceived effectiveness*: Even though they may feel it is important, clinicians generally feel ill-prepared to provide effective physical activity counseling.[8–11] Many clinicians cite lack of training as one of their most important barriers to counseling.[12] It is the unusual medical school or primary care residency, nursing, or other allied health professional program that provides training in behavior counseling. In part, this is due to the "medical model" approach so common to health professions education. Additionally, the science of behavioral medicine is relatively new, and many clinicians currently in practice trained before there was an established knowledge base in this area.
2. *Lack of time*: One of the most important issues for clinicians, and one of the most commonly cited barriers, is finding the time for behavior change counseling.[13] The relative shortage of primary care clinicians over the past decade has not lessened this problem.
3. *Lack of reimbursement*: The traditional fee-for-service structure of the health care marketplace has limited reimbursement for so-called cognitive interventions like counseling. The move toward managed care and other forms of prepaid health care is changing this situation and may even produce an environment in which health outcomes are valued more than procedures.
4. *Lack of standardized recommendations*: The absence of standardized recommendations both for the amount of physical activity individuals need and for approaches toward counseling[14] has created other barriers. The former problem has recently been addressed through the recent CDC–American College of Sports medicine recommendations on physical activity for adults.[15]

The PACE system was developed to address each of these issues. It is a relatively simple and easy-to-learn approach to physical activity counseling. It was designed to fit into a busy clinician's workday by being both quick to use (2 to 5 min) and adaptable to office practices, so that support staff can perform some, if not most, PACE functions. Given the quickness with which they can be used, the PACE materials can be cost-effective. And, because they standardize the approach to this issue, the materials reduce to a set of protocols for systematic counseling on a subject heretofore sometimes puzzling to clinicians. PACE materials include an explanatory *Physician's Manual, Assessment and Counseling Protocols*, as described below, progress note *Stickers* for medical charts, and a quick-review *Poster* for office or exam room use.

OVERVIEW OF PACE

The PACE program enables clinicians to address the modifiable determinants of physical activity such as self-efficacy, social support, and perceived barriers to action.[16] PACE enables clinicians to systematically use state-of-the-art behavioral counseling methods such as goal setting, barriers and solutions identification, contracting, social support network development, and self-efficacy improvement. With a little practice, the give-and-take embodied in the PACE approach becomes as natural as any other systematic approach to clinical information gathering and dissemination (Figure 3-1).

Before the patient sees the clinician, a *PACE Assessment Form* is completed. This form has been designed to be completed in less than 1 min and to need minimal explanation. On the front side of this form (Figure 3-2a) patients are asked to choose 1 of 11 graded statements that best describes their current level and interest and/or involvement in physical activity. The "grade" associated with each of these statements determines which of three "stages of change" (discussed more fully below) the patient is in. The back of the *PACE Assessment Form* (Figure 3-2b) contains the Physical Activity Readiness Questionnaire (PAR-Q), widely used in the physical activity and exercise counseling community as a method of screening for risk factors prior to beginning an activity program.[17]

After completing the questions on the Assessment Form, the patient returns it to the front-office staff and, based on their PACE score, is given one of three *PACE Counseling Protocols*:

Score 1—"Getting Out of Your Chair" for *Precontemplators* (Figures 3-3a and 3-3b)
Score 2 to 5—"Planning the First Step" for *Contemplators* (Figures 3-4a and 3-4b)
Score 6 to 11—"Keeping the PACE" for *Actives* (Figures 3-5a and 3-5b)

The patient takes 2 to 3 min to complete part of the front of the Counseling Protocol prior to seeing the clinician. With this information in hand, the clinician can then counsel the patient appropriately and make brief, individualized recommendations. The form also can serve as a prompt for clinician–patient dialogue about issues critical to adoption or maintenance of physical activity. The back of each protocol contains information and worksheets intended for patient use at home, with information that reinforces the physician's recommendations and ad-

PACE Assessment and Counseling Flow Chart

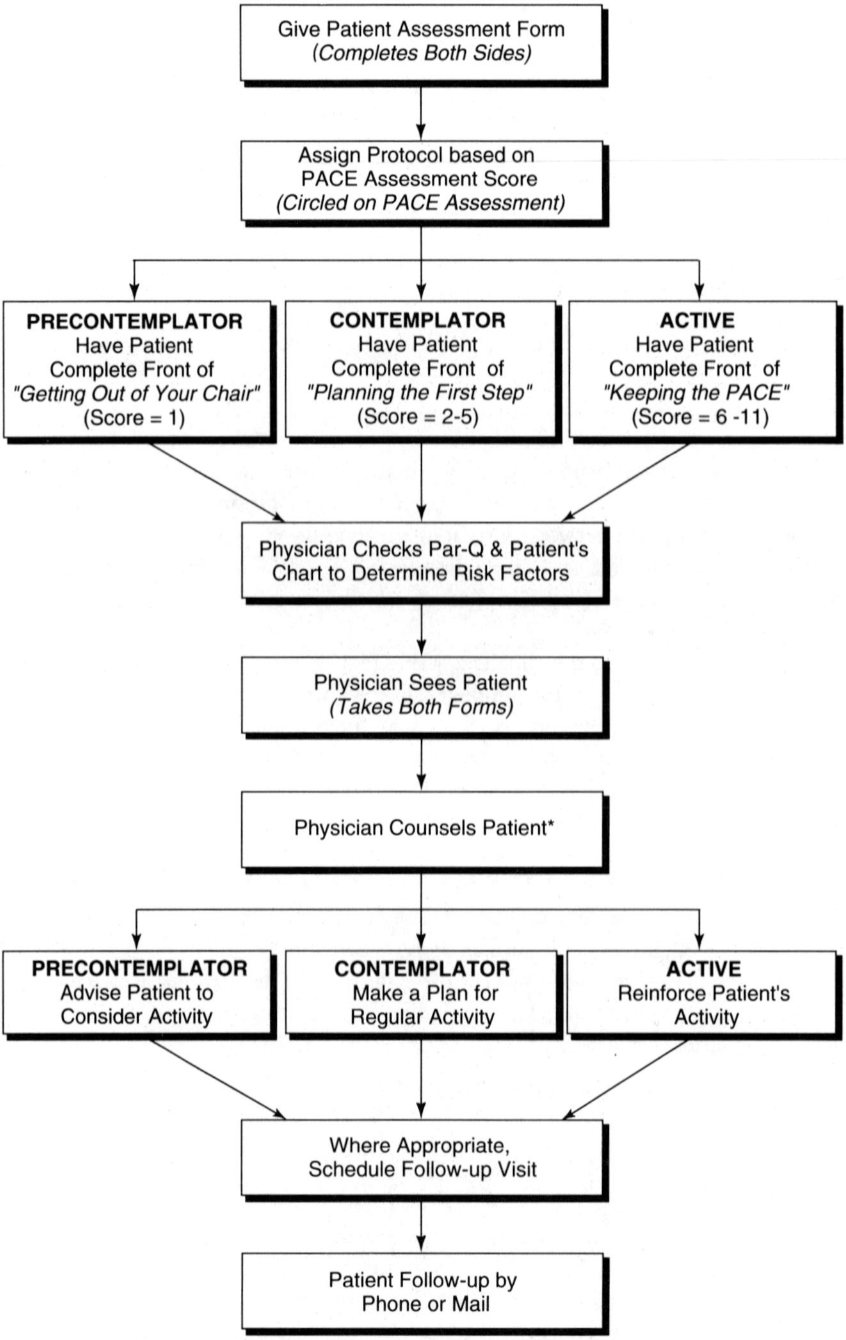

**Physician May Emphasize Importance of Physical Activity & Refer Patient to Other Health Care Professional in the Office for Counseling*

FIGURE 3-1. The overall structure of the PACE approach.

dresses stage-specific issues. The patient is given a copy of the counseling protocol and worksheet. A second copy may be kept in the medical record for documentation, for reminder purposes during the next visit, or for office staff use to determine which patients may benefit from follow-up procedures such as a phone call from the office staff and/or a post card. Postvisit techniques are recommended because they have been used successfully to enhance clinical interventions for dietary change[18] and physical activity change.[19]

THEORETICAL BASIS FOR PACE

Part of the PACE approach is based on contemporary knowledge about why people do or do not engage in physical activity.[16,20–22] Because knowledge and general attitudes about physical activity are not important influences, the PACE approach does not advocate trying to change these variables. Instead, PACE targets social and psychological factors known to influence physical activity, including social support, self-efficacy (or confidence that one can be active), perceived barriers, and awareness of the personal benefits of physical activity.[23] These factors are the most consistent correlates and predictors of physical activity, and each is targeted in the PACE intervention using a self-management approach.

Another aspect of PACE is that it aims to match the message the clinician gives to the one the patient is ready to hear. One counseling strategy is not appropriate for all patients. This understanding is embodied in the concept of the *stages of change*, which classifies patients according to their readiness to consider, adopt, or maintain a given behavior. Their readiness to do so is the essence of this approach and permits the synchronization of clinician guidance to patient acceptance.[24,25] People make behavioral change progressively, in stages, and have different counseling needs at each stage. Identifying the correct stage allows the provider to tailor a recommendation to the needs of the patient and use time effectively. The three PACE counseling protocols correspond to these stages of change: *Precontemplators, Contemplators, and Actives.*

Precontemplators are patients who are not active and, at the time of the clinical visit, have no intention or interest in beginning an activity program. The challenge for the clinician is to get precontemplators to consider beginning an activity program. These may be the kinds of patients who think physical activity and exercise is for the Jane Fondas and Arnold Swarzeneggers of the world but not for them. The approach taken in the "Getting Out of Your Chair" protocol is to ask them to identify *potential* personal benefits of physical activity. Patients are also asked to identify the two main reasons they're inactive and two ways they could overcome these roadblocks. The simple aim of this approach is to get these individuals to contemplate the value of physical activity and the potential benefits of it for them. The clinician can add his or her own suggestions about potential benefits for this person, depending on knowledge of the patient's health status. This process also sets the stage for the clinician to suggest potential ways to get around roadblocks.

Clinicians should not spend time suggesting a beginner's physical activity plan. Rather, they should acknowledge patients' choice *not* to be active now but remain

Patient's Name ____________ Date ______

What is Your PACE SCORE?

This form will help your doctor understand your level of physical activity. Please read the entire form and then choose the number below that best describes your *current* level of physical activity or your interest in physical activity. Do *not* include activities that you do as part of your job.

"Vigorous" exercise includes activities like jogging, running, fast cycling, aerobics classes, swimming laps, singles tennis, and racquetball. Any activity that makes you work *as hard as jogging* and lasts *20 minutes* at a time should be counted. These types of activities usually increase your heart rate, and make you sweat, and you get out of breath. *(Do not count weight lifting.)*

"Moderate" exercise includes activities like brisk walking, gardening, slow cycling, dancing, doubles tennis, or hard work around the house. Any activity that makes you work *as hard as brisk walking* and that lasts at least *30 minutes* at a time should be counted.

Circle One Number Only	*CURRENT PHYSICAL ACTIVITY STATUS*
1.	I do not exercise or walk regularly now, and I do not intend to start in the near future.
2.	I do not exercise or walk regularly, but I have been thinking of starting.
3.	I am trying to start to exercise or walk. *(or)* During the last month I have started to exercise or walk on occasion *(or on weekends only)*.
4.	I have exercised or walked infrequently *(or on weekends only)* for over one month.
5.	I am doing vigorous or moderate exercise, less than 3 times per week *(or moderate exercise less than 2 hours per week)*.
6.	I have been doing moderate exercise, 3 or more times per week *(or more than 2 hours per week)* for the last 1-6 months.
7.	I have been doing moderate exercise, 3 or more times per week *(or more than 2 hours per week)* for 7 months or more.
8.	I have been doing vigorous exercise, 3-5 times per week for 1-6 months.
9.	I have been doing vigorous exercise, 3-5 times per week for 7-12 months.
10.	I have been doing vigorous exercise, 3-5 times per week for over 12 months.
11.	I do vigorous exercise 6 or more times per week.

rev 11/92

Please Complete Other Side

FIGURE 3-2a.

interested and available should these patients change their minds. This approach sends a clear, personal message to the patients but does not turn them off to the idea of physical activity. The door is open for further discussion.

The approach to *Precontemplators* can be summarized as follows:

- Summarize the benefits of exercise.
- Relate the benefits to the patient's personal health status.
- Have the patient list personal reasons to be active.
- Have the patient identify barriers to physical activity.

*PHYSICAL ACTIVITY READINESS QUESTIONNAIRE (PAR-Q)**

A SELF-ADMINISTERED QUESTIONAIRRE FOR ADULTS

PAR-Q is designed to help you help yourself. Many health benefits are associated with regular exercise, and the completion of PAR-Q is a sensible first step to take if you are planning to increase the amount of physical activity in your life.

For most people, physical activity should not pose any problem or hazard. PAR-Q has been designed to identify the small number of adults for whom physical activity might be inappropriate or those who should have medical advice concerning the type of activity most suitable for them.

Common sense is your best guide in answering these questions. Please read them carefully and check YES or NO opposite the question as it applies to you.

YES	NO		
☐	☐	1.	Has a doctor ever said that you have a heart condition and recommended only medically supervised activity?
☐	☐	2.	Do you have chest pain brought on by physical activity?
☐	☐	3.	Have you developed chest pain in the past month?
☐	☐	4.	Do you tend to lose consciousness or fall over as a result of dizziness?
☐	☐	5.	Do you have a bone or joint problem that could be aggravated by the proposed physical activity?
☐	☐	6.	Has a doctor ever recommended medication for your high blood pressure or a heart condition?
☐	☐	7.	Are you aware through your own experience, or a doctor's advice, of any other physical reason against your exercising without medical supervision?

Note: *If you have a temporary illness, such as a common cold, or are not feeling well at this time --* ***Postpone.***

You are participating in a national program that is designed to increase physical activity among adults. We need to know what you think of the information you receive from your healthcare providers today. If you would be willing to talk to a researcher over the telephone in the near future, please sign below and give us a phone number and time of day that you prefer to be called. *Thank you for your help.*

FIGURE 3-2b.

- Give clear advice to consider a physical activity program.

Contemplators are patients who do little or no regular physical activity, are aware of the need to do so, and are "thinking about it." people in this group often need the knowledge, skills, or right kind of encouragement to become active. The goal of the "Planning the First Step" protocol is just that: to help the patient make a specific plan to begin an activity program. Counseling begins with positive feedback to patients for their desire to become active. In addition to identifying the benefits of their activity program, these patients draft a brief activity plan which they review with the clinician, including what, where, and when they will do it. Finally, they

____________________ ________

Patient's Name Date

GETTING OUT OF YOUR CHAIR

On your PACE Assessment you said that you are not very interested in physical activity. Have you thought very much about what *you* can get out of being active?

- *Physical Activity can help you feel better*
- *Physical Activity can help you look better*
- *Physical Activity can help you be healthier*

What would be the two most important benefits of physical activity *for you*? Be specific.

1. ____

2. ____

Do you know you can get most of the benefits of physical activity just by *walking* on a regular basis? You do not have to jog or go to aerobics classes to be an exerciser.

Many things can interfere with physical activity. Here are some of the reasons people give for not being physically active. Check the ones that apply most to you.

______ Exercise is hard work
______ I am usually too tired for exercise
______ I do not have anyone to exercise with me
______ The weather is too bad
______ There is no convenient place
______ I am too overweight
______ I do not enjoy exercise
______ I hate to fail, so I will not start
______ I do not have a safe place to exercise
______ Exercise is boring
______ I do not have the time
______ I am too old

What are the two main things that keep you from wanting to be physically active?

1. ____

2. ____

The good news is you can do something about the reasons you are not physically active. If you think of them as *roadblocks* between you and physical activity, you can figure out how to get around them. You can change the roadblock itself *(I will get up earlier in the morning to make time for physical activity).* You can also change your attitude about the roadblock *(I really can find some time to exercise).*

How can you get around your two main roadblocks? Look at the ideas on the back of this sheet.

1. ____

2. ____

THE FIRST STEP IN BEING PHYSICALLY ACTIVE IS GETTING OUT OF YOUR CHAIR.

Provider's Use Only:

Based on your health status, your doctor recommends you do the following to improve your health:

______ You appear to be able to do either moderate or vigorous physical activities.
______ You can benefit greatly by starting a program of regular walking or other moderate activity. If you want to do activities as hard as jogging, you need to have an exercise tolerance test.*
______ Before you increase your physical activity, you need to have an exercise tolerance test.*

**Call this office for an appointment or referral.*

____
Provider's Signature

rev 11/92

FIGURE 3-3a.

are asked to identify a family member, friend, or coworker who will support their new activity program. The more specific patients can be regarding the details of their program, the more likely they will be able to adhere to it.

Based on the information provided by patients—and on their past medical history and current health status—the clinician reinforces the plan of activity and addresses

Your physician strongly encourages you to:
- think about the benefits you can get from physical activity and
- think about how you can avoid some of the roadblocks between you and physical activity.

Most people can improve their health a great deal by taking a walk for 30 minutes 3-4 times every week. If you want information on how to start doing more physical activity, ask your doctor.

BENEFITS OF PHYSICAL ACTIVITY

☆ *IMPROVE YOUR HEALTH*
- Reduce your risk of *heart disease*
- Reduce your risk of some kinds of *cancer*
- Reduce your risk of *diabetes*
- Strengthen your *bones*

☆ *INCREASE YOUR ENERGY*

☆ *MAINTAIN OR LOSE WEIGHT*

☆ *IMPROVE YOUR MOOD AND SELF-ESTEEM. FEEL BETTER ABOUT YOURSELF.*

HOW TO GET PAST ROADBLOCKS

ROADBLOCK:	HOW TO GET PAST IT:
_____ Exercise is hard work	Pick an activity that you enjoy and that is easy for you. "No pain, no gain" is a myth.
_____ I do not have time	We're only talking about three 30 minute sessions each week. Can you do without three TV shows each week?
_____ I do not enjoy exercise	Do not "exercise." Start a hobby or way of playing that gets you moving.
_____ I am usually too tired to exercise	Tell yourself, "This activity will give me more energy." See if it doesn't happen.
_____ I do not have a safe place to exercise	If your neighborhood is not safe, you can walk at work, walk in a group, or walk in the morning.
_____ I do not have anyone to exercise with me	Maybe you have not asked. A neighbor, family member or co-worker may be a willing partner. Or you can choose an activity that you enjoy doing by yourself.
_____ There is no convenient place	Pick an activity you can do near your home or work. Walk around your neighborhood or do aerobics with a TV show at home.
_____ I am afraid of being injured	Walking is very safe, and it is an excellent activity to improve your health.
_____ The weather is too bad	There are many activities you can do in your home, in any weather.
_____ Exercise is boring	Listening to music during your activity keeps your mind occupied. Walking, biking, or running can take you past lots of interesting scenery.
_____ I am too overweight	You can benefit from physical activity regardless of your weight. Pick an activity that you are comfortable with, like walking.
_____ I am too old	It's never too late to start. If you are ill, it is important to talk to your doctor about physical activity.

FIGURE 3-3b.

barriers. Both the patient and physician agree to a "contracted program" for a specified period of time and sign an agreement. This approach has been shown to be an effective behavioral modification technique. Although counseling these patients is the most time-consuming of the three stages, with practice counseling should take no more than 5 min. Also, these are the patients most likely to make the greatest gains in physical activity; therefore, it is appropriate to spend the most

______________________ ________

Patient's Name Date

PLANNING THE FIRST STEP

Congratulations. On your PACE Assessment you said that you arc ready to make physical activity a regular part of your life. You are taking a big step toward improving your physical and mental health. This form should be able to help you start an activity program you can stick with.

What are the two main benefits you hope to get from being active? Write them down here and think of them often.

1. ______________________ 2. ______________________

PHYSICAL ACTIVITY MUST BE REGULAR. Plan to do an activity of your choice, 3-5 times per week.

WHAT ACTIVITIES ARE YOU GOING TO DO?

Some activities enjoyed by many people are listed on the back. In choosing *your* activity, consider these questions:

- **Do you enjoy it?** Can you afford the supplies, equipment, facilities, or classes? Are there family or friends to do this activity with you? Can you do it year-round or do you need more than one activity?
  *Type(s) of Activity:*______________________
- **Where will you do your activity?** Can you do this activity at home or in your neighborhood? Do you have to go to a gym, a park, or a health club? Is this place convenient for you?
  Place(s) for Activity: ______________________
- **What is the most realistic time for you to do this activity 3 to 5 times per week?** Will you have to reschedule other activities?
  Days and Times for Activity: ______________________
- **How long to you plan to do your activity each time?** Build up time gradually over several weeks. Start with a 5-10 minute workout and build up to 30-60 minutes of moderate activity or 20-40 minutes of vigorous activity.
  *Length of Activity:*______________________
- **Who can support you or help with your new activity program?** It is ideal for someone to be active with you. You may want to ask someone to encourage you or help you to be active.
  *Who will help you, and how?*______________________

Provider's Use Only:

Based on your health status, your doctor recommends you do the following to improve your health:

_____ You appear to be able to do either moderate or vigorous physical activities.

_____ You can benefit greatly by starting a program of regular walking or other moderate activity. If you want to do activities as hard as jogging, you need to have an exercise tolerance test.*

_____ Before you increase your physical activity, you need to have an exercise tolerance test.*

**Call this office for an appointment or referral.*

SUGGESTED PROGRAM (FITT)

Frequency F _____ times per week
Intensity I _____ moderate _____ vigorous activity
Type T _____ type of physical activity
Time T _____ minutes per session to begin
[work up to ___ min. in ___ weeks.]

MAJOR CVD RISK FACTORS

☐ Smoking
☐ Hypertension
☐ Elevated Lipids
☐ Physical Inactivity
☐ Positive Family History

*I agree to try out this physical activity plan from:*______________ *to:*______________

______________________ ______________________

Patient's Signature Provider's Signature

rev 11/92

FIGURE 3-4a.

time with them. Once prompted by the clinician, these patients can be referred to office support and/or health educational staff for more detailed and extensive counseling. It may also be helpful to provide additional written materials, many of which are available through local and national organizations.

The approach to *Contemplators* can be summarized as follows:

- Praise the patient.

ACTIVITIES

MODERATE:	**VIGOROUS**
Walking (at home, to work, on lunch break)	*Jogging*
Gardening (must be regular)	*Aerobic dance*
Hiking	*Basketball*
Slow cycling	*Fast Cycling*
Folk, square, or popular dancing	*Cross-country skiing*
Ice and roller skating	*Swimming laps*
Doubles tennis	*Singles tennis and racquet sports*
Taking the stairs	*Soccer*

HOW TO GET PAST ROADBLOCKS

ROADBLOCK:	**HOW TO GET PAST IT:**
_____ I do not have the time	We're only talking about three 30-minute sessions each week. Can you do without three TV shows each week?
_____ I do not enjoy exercise	Do not "exercise." Start a hobby or an enjoyable activity that gets you moving.
_____ I am usually too tired to exercise	Regular activity will *improve* your energy level. Try it and see for yourself!
_____ The weather is too bad	There are many activities you can do in your own home, in any weather.
_____ Exercise is boring	Listening to music during your activity keeps your mind occupied. Walking, biking, or running can take you past lots of interesting scenery.
_____ I get sore when I exercise	Slight muscle soreness after physical activity is common when you are just starting. It should go away in 2-3 days. You can avoid this by building up gradually and stretching after the activity.

ACTIVITY LOG

Use this Activity Log to keep track of your physical activity. Write down how long you do your activity as well as positive feelings and experiences. Note any roadblocks that discourage you from doing your activity and do something about them. When this log is full, make one of your own.

Date	Activity	Minutes	Feelings/Comments

Good Luck and Keep Moving!

FIGURE 3-4b.

- Give clear advice to begin a physical activity program.
- Have the patient identify the benefits he or she hopes to obtain from physical activity.
- Have the patient choose a preferred and appropriate activity.
- Have the patient identify sources of social support.
- Have the patient identify barriers to physical activity.

____________________ ________

Patient's Name Date

KEEPING THE PACE

Congratulations. You are doing regular physical activity. You have a right to feel proud that you are doing something very positive for yourself. Sometimes you may lose sight of the physical and mental health benefits you are getting from physical activity. What motivates you to stay active?

1) __________ 2) __________ 3) __________

REVIEW YOUR PROGRAM

By reviewing the activities you are doing now, you can see if any changes need to be made in your plan. The goal is to improve your chances of *staying* active.

What *type(s)* of activity do you usually do? __________
How many *times a week*? __________
How long each time? __________
Who *helps* you or does the activity with you? __________
Have you had any *injuries*? __________
What parts of your activity plan are you *most satisfied* with? __________
What parts of your activity plan are you *least satisfied* with? __________
What *changes* might you make in your activity plan to make it more enjoyable, convenient, or safe? __________

GETTING BACK ON TRACK

Most people who are regularly active have stopped at one time or another in the past. Sometimes they stop for a few weeks. Sometimes it is years before they start being active again. Planning ahead by answering these questions now can help you get past roadblocks later.

- If you have stopped regular activity in the past, what caused you to stop? __________
- What could you have done differently that would have helped you stay active or what helped you to get back on track quickly? __________

KEEPING THE PACE

How confident are you that you can continue to do regular physical activity for the next 3 months?

(Please circle) NO CONFIDENCE LOW CONFIDENCE MEDIUM CONFIDENCE HIGH CONFIDENCE

What is reducing your confidence and what can you do to improve it? __________

Provider's Use Only:

SUMMARY OF CURRENT PROGRAM (FITT)

Frequency F ____ times per week
Intensity I ____ moderate ____ vigorous activity
Type T ____ type of physical activity
Time T ____ minutes per session to begin
[work up to ____ min. in ____ weeks.]

MAJOR CVD RISK FACTORS

☐ Smoking
☐ Hypertension
☐ Elevated Lipids
☐ Physical Inactivity
☐ Positive Family History

____
Provider's Signature

rev 11/92

FIGURE 3-5a.

- Have the patient rate his or her confidence in being able to do regular physical activity.
- Patient and clinician sign a contract for physical activity.
- Schedule a follow-up appointment.
- Reward patient with praise.

Actives are just that—patients active at a level sufficient to gain the benefits of

TIPS FOR KEEPING THE PACE

Injury to muscle, joints and bones may be the *most common* cause of stopping activity. The best way to prevent injury is to start gradually. Do not do an activity that is too vigorous for you. If you are overdoing it, slow down. If you feel pain during physical activity, stop and rest. The ***most serious*** risk of physical activity is heart trouble, but it is *rare*. If you feel pain in your chest, immediately stop the activity and consult a physician.

The PACE recommendation of 30 to 60 minutes of moderate activity or 20 to 40 minutes of vigorous activity provides maximum benefit at low levels of risk. Exercise scientists also suggest warming up before your main activity and cooling down and stretching after your activity to lower your risk of injury. Warming up and cooling down can be slow versions of your activity, like slow walking. Gently stretch the muscles you use during the activity. Hold each stretch 5-10 seconds and don't bounce.

There are times when you may stop your regular activity. This may be due to more demands on your time at home or work, travel, house guests, or illness. Interruptions are normal and expected. ***The key is starting your regular activity again as soon as possible.***

LOOK AHEAD FOR YOUR ROADBLOCKS

What situation or thing is most likely to make you stop being active?____________________

____

What can you do about this roadblock to prevent it or prepare for it? ____________________

____

What is the best way for you to get back on track if you stop? ____________________

____

HOW TO GET BACK ON TRACK

- Remind yourself it is okay to have a pause in your activity once in a while. Don't be hard on yourself. Feeling guilty will make it more difficult to get back on track.
- You may need some extra help to get going again. Ask family and friends to help and encourage you.
- Ask someone to exercise with you.
- It may be helpful to tell everybody you know that you are restarting your activity plan.
- Use an Activity Log to keep track of your activity again.
- Give yourself small rewards each time you do your physical activity. Make a chart for your refrigerator. Use stickers or gold stars to keep track of your activity. Put change in a jar as a reward. Praising yourself is an effective reward *("I did it and I'm proud of myself!")*.
- For variety, try new activities.
- Do whatever worked for you in the past to restart physical activity.

FIGURE 3-5b.

regular physical activity. The clinician's counseling goal for actives is to keep them active and to help them anticipate how to maintain physical activity as their health and life progress. Counseling these patients begins by congratulating them on their active lives. Praise can be a powerful motivator. Patients should be asked to identify the benefits they receive from their activity, and to review their current program and consider any changes which might make it more enjoyable. Occasional periods of inactivity (relapse) for avoidable or unavoidable reasons are expected, and long-term adherence is dependent on one's skill in getting back on track quickly. Clinicians should outline strategies for preventing relapse and returning to activity. Finally, clinicians should ask patients how confident they are that they will maintain their activity program for the next 3 months. This is a measure of physical activity self-efficacy and a good indicator of future success. The counseling ends as the physician summarizes the mutually agreed-on plan and both the physician and the patient sign an exercise contract.

The approach to *Actives* can be summarized as follows:

- Reward the patient with praise.
- Review the current physical activity program.
- Have the patient identify sources of social support for *regular* activity.
- Have the patient identify barriers to regular activity or to resumption of activity following periods of relapse.
- Have the patient develop solutions to barriers.
- Have the patient rate his or her confidence in being able to continue regular physical activity.
- Schedule a follow-up appointment.

For all three of these patient groups, the most important counseling skills are *giving specific advice, setting realistic goals, joint problem solving* to overcome barriers, and ensuring *positive reinforcement* of success to boost confidence. An example of the use of the PACE materials is given in the following case example.

CASE EXAMPLE

A Clinician's Encounter With a Contemplator

Mrs. Diego is a 55-year-old woman who works as a secretary in a shipyard. She has three children (28, 25, and 22 years old). Her husband died of a heart attack 2 years ago. She is being seen for her annual physical examination, and acknowledges feeling stressed at home and at work. She indicates on her Contemplator protocol that she would like to be active to (1) lose weight and (2) decrease stress. She used to walk with her husband after dinner and would like to start walking again three or four times per week.

Medical History: Nonsmoker; medications: estrogen replacement therapy.

Review of Systems: No chest pain, SOB, pedal edema, or CNS symptoms.

Family Medical History: Father died at age 70 of heart attack; otherwise unremarkable.

Physical Exam: BP 110/80, height 5′3″, weight 150 lb. The rest of the exam was WNL.

Lab Findings: Cholesterol 250 mg/dl. Triglycerides WNL.

Activity History: Not very active as a youth. Used to walk with her husband 3–4 times a week after dinner.

PACE Score: 2: "I used to exercise or walk regularly; I am thinking about starting." *Preliminary Assessment*: Risk factors: soft family history of CHD, hypercholesterolemia, approximately 20% over ideal body weight (130 lb for medium frame), and currently has a sedentary lifestyle. In addition, she feels stressed. No contraindications to beginning a moderate physical activity program.

MD: Mrs. Diego, I see you used to walk with your husband on a regular basis. Why did you stop?

Mrs. Diego: After Sam died, I didn't have the desire. My youngest daughter is encouraging me to become more active, though. I guess I'm ready to get started again.

MD: That's great! The two benefits of starting a physical activity program that you've listed on your PACE form are good ones. With moderate physical activity, and of course a proper diet, you can lose weight and keep it off. Plus, you can feel better about yourself. Based on your lab work, your cholesterol is elevated. Physical activity, along with cutting down on your dietary cholesterol and fats, may help improve this. So, decreased cholesterol is another reason to get back into walking. I'd like to get a fasting lipid profile to look a little further into this.

Mrs. Diego: That sounds good. Do I need to worry about a heart attack like Sam's? How do I get started?

MD: A heart attack isn't very likely for you. A specific plan is the key to successful physical activity. You used to enjoy walking—an excellent choice for now since it's been a couple of years since you've been very active, but you might want to start out with two times per week. Begin at slow pace. Do you feel comfortable starting out with about 15 minutes?

Mrs. Diego: Yes.

MD: Good. By not overdoing it, you also reduce the risk of a muscle or joint injury. Gradually increase by 5 minutes a week until you reach 45 or 60 minutes a session. If it's convenient, you can walk during your lunch break and take the stairs instead of the elevator. I see you listed Wednesday's at lunch time and Mondays and Fridays after dinner as good times for you. How confident are you that you can walk 15 minutes on two of those days?

Mrs. Diego: I know I can do that. I'm relieved. I thought you were going to tell me to do it every day, and I don't think I could do that. I'll ask my daughter to walk with me. But doctor, how fast should I walk?

MD: At first, nice and easy. Eventually, you'll want to be able to carry on a conversation with your daughter while walking briskly enough to perspire a bit. You should purchase some good supportive walking shoes. I have a handout to help you pick out some good ones.

Mrs. Diego: Well, I'm confident I can get started! I'm glad you brought this up.

MD: Great! To summarize: your program will consist of walking two times a week at a moderate stride for 15 minutes to begin the first week. Gradually increase 5 to 10 minutes a week until you reach 45 minutes total. Let your body be your guide. If you agree with this, just sign this agreement, and I'll sign too. This is our way of making a commitment to trying this plan for 2 weeks. Here is your copy. On the back are some other examples of moderate physical activity; some barriers to physical activity and ways to get around them; and a log to record your physical activity sessions. Put this somewhere where you can see it—for example, on your refrigerator. If you have any problems, don't hesitate to call. I'd like to see you in 6 weeks to recheck your cholesterol and review your progress. And I'll ask the nurse to discuss dietary habits with you. See you in a few weeks!

SUMMARY

1. The PACE system guides the clinician and patient as they engage in brief, personalized negotiations about physical activity. Based on the latest research in primary care, exercise science, and the behavioral sciences, PACE is a structured, reproducible, and efficacious health promotion tool.[26] As such, it represents the kind of health promotion tool we anticipate seeing more of in the future.
2. PACE is based on determining the "stage of change" of a patient with respect to the intent to become physically active. Once this stage—precontemplation, contemplation or active—is determined, specific guidance for negotiation between clinician and patient is enabled and supported, and the clinician doesn't waste time discussing topics that are not relevant to the patient.
3. PACE is currently being considered for adaptation to populations other than its initial target group, apparently healthy adults. Children, the frail elderly, certain ethnic minority groups, and others may have special needs to address within the PACE approach. As these are developed and evaluated, they will be reported in the primary care literature. The PACE team welcomes any and all suggestions for the improvement of this exciting means of getting and keeping patients active.

Acknowledgment

PACE was developed with the support of the U.S. Public Health Service, Centers for Disease Control and Prevention. The views in this chapter do not necessarily represent those of the U.S. Public Health Service.

For information about ordering PACE materials, or about continuing research and development activities for PACE, contact: Project PACE, San Diego State University, Student Health Services, 5500 Campanile Drive, San Diego, California 92182-4701 or call 619-594-5949.

REFERENCES

1. *Healthy People 2000: National Health Promotion and Disease Prevention Objectives*. Pub. No. (PHS) 91-50213. Washington, DC: U.S. Public Health Service, U.S. Department of Health and Human Services, 1991.
2. Caspersen CJ, Christenson GM, Pollard RA: Status of the 1990 physical fitness

and exercise objectives-evidence from NHIS 1985. *Public Health Rep* 101:587–592, 1986.

3. A new tool for encouraging activity: Project PACE. *Physician Sportsmed* 22(11):45–55, 1994.
4. Weaver FJ, Herrick KL, Ramirez AG, et al: Establishing a community base for a cardiovascular health education program. *Health Values* 2:249–256, 1978.
5. American College of Sports Medicine: *Guidelines for Exercise Testing and Exercise Prescription*, ed 3. Philadelphia, Lea and Febiger, 1986.
6. Wells KB, Ware JE, Lewis CE: Physicians' practices in counseling patients about health habits. *Med Care* 22:240–246, 1984.
7. Mullen P, Tabak GR: Patterns of counseling techniques used by family practice physicians for smoking, weight, exercise, and stress. *Med Care* 27:694–704, 1989.
8. Wells KB, Lewis CE, Leake B, et al: The practice of general and subspecialty internists in counseling about smoking and exercise. *Am J Health* 76:1009–1013, 1986.
9. Mullen PD, Tabak ER: Patterns of counseling techniques used by family practice physicians for smoking, weight, exercise and stress. *Med Care* 27:694–704, 1989.
10. Lewis CE, Clancy C, Leake B, et al: The counseling practices of internists. *Ann Intern Med* 114:54–58, 1991.
11. Orleans CT, George LK, Houpt JL, et al: Health promotion in primary care: A survey of U.S. family practitioners. *Prev Med* 14:636–647, 1985.
12. Wells KB, Lewis CE, Leake B, et al: Do physicians preach what they practice? A study of physicians' health habits and counseling practices. *JAMA* 252:2846–2848, 1986.
13. National Center for Health Statistics: *Health, United States, 1990*. Hyattsville, Md.: U.S. Public Health Service, 1990.
14. Johns MB, Hovell MF, Ganiats T, et al: Primary care and health promotion: A model for preventive medicine. *Am J Prev Med* 3:346–357, 1987.
15. Pate RR, Pratt M, Blair SN, et al: Physical activity and public health, a recommendation from the Centers for Disease Control and Prevention and the American College of Sports Medicine. *JAMA* 273(5):402–407, 1995.
16. Sallis JF, Hovell MF: Determinants of exercise behavior. *Exerc Sports Sci Rev* 18:307–330, 1990.
17. Shephard RJ: PAR-Q, Canadian Home Fitness Test and exercise screening alternatives. *Sports Med* 5:185–195, 1988.
18. Crouch M, Sallis JF, Farquhar JW, et al: Personal and mediated health counseling for sustained dietary reduction of hypercholesterolemia. *Prev Med* 15:282–291, 1986.
19. Owen N, Lee C, Naccarella L, et al: Exercise by mail: A mediated behavior-change program for aerobic exercise. *J Sport Psych* 9:346–357, 1987.
20. Dishman RK: Determinants of participation in physical activity. In Bouchard C, Shephard RJ, Stephens T, et al (eds): *Exercise, Fitness, and Health: A Consensus of Current Knowledge*. Champaign, Ill, Human Kinetics, 1990, pp 75–102.
21. Sallis JF, Hovell MF, Hofstetter CR, et al: Explanation of vigorous physical activity during two years using social learning variables. *Soc Sci Med* 34:25–32, 1991.
22. Sallis JF, Hovell MF, Hofstetter CR: Predictors of adoption and maintenance of vigorous physical activity in men and women. *Prev Med* 21:237–251, 1992.
23. Dishman RK, Sallis JF: Determinants and interventions for physical activity and exercise. In Bouchard C, Shephard RJ, Stephens T (eds): *Physical Activity, Fitness and Health: International Proceedings and Consensus Statement*. Champaign, Ill, Human Kinetics, 1994, pp 214–238.
24. Prochaska JO, DiClemente CC: Stages and processes of self-change of smoking: Toward

an integrative model of change. *Journal of Consulting and Clinical Psychology* 51:390–395, 1983.

25. Marcus BH, Banspach SW, Lefebvre RC, et al: Using the stages of change model to increase the adoption of physical activity among community participants. *Am J Health Promotion* 6:424–429, 1992.
26. Calfas KJ, Long BJ, Sallis JF, et al. A controlled trial of physician counseling to promote the adoption of physical activity. *Prev Med* (in press).

• CHAPTER FOUR •

THE PREPARTICIPATION EXAMINATION

Mary C. Fahrenbach, M.D.
Randal J. Thomas, M.D., M.S.

CASE EXAMPLE

Patient History and Examination

You are asked to perform a preparticipation examination on a 19-year-old college freshman who is trying out for her school's soccer team. She reports no current or previous problems with her health. She mentions that she has been told in the past by several doctors that she has a heart murmur, but that it is not something about which she should worry. On physical examination her blood pressure is 110/64 mm Hg in the right arm (average of three readings) and 114/60 mm Hg in the left arm. Systolic blood pressure in the lower extremities is 126 mm Hg on the right and 128 mm Hg on the left. The radial pulse is strong and is not biphasic. No delay is noted when comparing the radial and femoral pulses simultaneously. A soft grade II/VI early systolic murmur is heard at the apex that does not radiate to the carotid arteries. The murmur nearly disappears on standing and during the early phase of Valsalva's maneuver. The heart's point of maximal impact (PMI) is nondisplaced and normal in character.

Comments/Questions

What are the possible diagnoses? Does the patient have an innocent murmur? Do you have enough information on which to base a decision on clearance for athletic participation? If so, what would your advice be? If not, what further information is necessary before the patient can be given advice regarding athletic participation?

INTRODUCTION

The preparticipation screening of persons involved in athletic activities has been advocated as a means to identify those individuals at risk for exercise-related cardiac complications. Unfortunately, there are limitations to this strategy since cardiac events occurring during and immediately after exercise are rare and physical findings predictive of increased risk during exercise are often lacking, particularly in people with underlying coronary artery disease (CAD). Nonetheless, the preparticipation physical examination is an essential prerequisite for athletic training. It also offers the physician a unique opportunity to meet with the patient-athlete and to discuss the health impacts of habitual physical activity and other lifestyle behaviors (e.g., cigarette smoking, diet, drug use, sexual activity, seat belt use, and bicycle safety helmet use).

CARDIOVASCULAR COMPLICATIONS OF EXERCISE

Strategies for the preparticipation screening of athletes should take into account the low risk of cardiovascular complications during exercise. One study found that the incidence of sudden death during jogging in Rhode Island among men aged 30 to 65 years was only one death per year for every 7620 joggers.[1] When men with known CAD were removed from the analysis, the risk of sudden cardiac death decreased to one death for every 15,240 joggers. Similarly, Siscovick et al.[2] found only one exercise-related cardiac arrest for every 18,000 men aged 25 to 75 years who had no prior history of CAD. There are no accurate data in these studies[1,2] on the incidence of nonfatal complications of exercise since these events were rarely reported.

The presence of underlying CAD does increase the risk of exercise-related sudden cardiac death (SCD). The death rate per hour of jogging in the general adult population is one per every 400,000 hours of activity.[1] In contrast, there is one cardiac arrest for every 33,000 to 112,000 hours of activity among patients involved in cardiac rehabilitation programs.[3,4] However, even among patients with

CAD, the incidence of fatal cardiac arrests is extremely low; only three were observed among 167 cardiac rehabilitation programs during approximately 2,350,000 hours of activity.[4] These figures may not be applicable to the general population with CAD since the patients who suffered an arrest in these reports presumably had ready access to resuscitation equipment. In populations with a low prevalence of CAD, such as persons under age 35 years, a much lower incidence of SCD is seen. For example, among U.S. Air Force recruits, only one death was observed for every 3,000,000 hours of exercise, or one death per every 735,000 men.[5] Again, these results are probably not applicable to all young people because military personnel are medically screened before induction into service.

There are very few data on the incidence of SCD among unselected populations of young people. There is even less information regarding the incidence of exercise-related cardiovascular events among women and minority groups. The yearly death rate during physical activity for a population of Rhode Island men under age 30 was one death for every 280,000 persons.[6] The denominator for this estimate, however, was all young men in Rhode Island and was not restricted to the subgroup who exercised. In this study,[6] no deaths were observed over 7 years among young women (age <29).

The studies described above underscore the principle that the incidence of exercise-related SCD and nonfatal cardiac events is low, especially in those populations with a low prevalence of CAD. Also, strategies aimed at screening persons who desire to exercise must emphasize the identification of risk factors for CAD.

CAUSES OF SCD

Atherosclerotic CAD is by far the most common cause of SCD, especially in individuals over age 35.[7,8] Among individuals aged 35 or less, structural cardiac abnormalities predominate as the most common conditions predisposing to SCD. The various causes of SCD are listed in Table 4-1. Maron et al.[9] evaluated a series of 29 cases of SCD in a population of young (age 13 to 30 years), competitive

TABLE 4-1. Causes of sudden death during exertion in young subjects

More Common	Less Common
Hypertrophic cardiomyopathy	Myocarditis
Anomalous coronary artery origin and course	Aortic stenosis
Atherosclerotic coronary artery disease	Mitral valve prolapse
Aortic rupture (Marfan syndrome)	Right ventricular dysplasia
Idiopathic concentric left ventricular hypertrophy	Conduction system abnormalities
	Amyloidosis
	Sarcoidosis
	Cardiac tumors

Source: Adapted from Ref. 15 with permission.

athletes and found that hypertrophic cardiomyopathy (HCM) was the most common underlying condition, accounting for 14 cases. Other causes of SCD in this series were idiopathic concentric left ventricular hypertrophy, which may represent a variant of HCM[8] (five cases), anomalous origin of the left coronary artery (three cases), atherosclerotic CAD (three cases), rupture of the aorta (two cases), and hypoplastic coronary arteries (one case). Interestingly, in one autopsy, the heart was reported to be completely normal.

Waller[10] reviewed a larger number of exercise-related deaths (72) occurring in persons aged 30 years or younger. In this series, the most common cause of SCD was congenital coronary anomalies (38 cases), predominantly an anomalous origin of the left main coronary artery from the right sinus of Valsalva, with an abnormal course between the aorta and the pulmonary trunk. The cause of death in this condition is probably the acute angle of take-off and the presence of ostial valve–like ridges in the anomalous artery which lead to sudden occlusion, especially if the artery is also compressed by a dilated aortic root.[11] Other causes of SCD in Waller's series included HCM (16 cases), atherosclerotic CAD (4 cases), mitral valve prolapse (2 cases), idiopathic dilated cardiomyopathy (1 case) and myocarditis (1 case). In 17 cases of SCD, the cause was believed to be "indeterminate" or "traumatic." Causes of SCD can also be specific to the population studied. In the review by Phillips et al.[5] of 19 cases of SCD among U.S. Air Force recruits, myocarditis was the most common underlying etiology (8 cases), followed by anomalous coronary arteries (3 cases), and HCM (2 cases). These authors speculate that in this special population, the relatively high incidence of myocarditis may relate to the uniform immunization of recruits early in training.

THE GENERAL PREPARTICIPATION PHYSICAL EXAMINATION

As outlined above, SCD during exercise is a rare event, even in older populations with documented CAD. Thus, screening programs to identify individuals at risk for SCD are by definition limited, since large populations must be examined to identify those few persons who are most likely to die. Furthermore, several conditions that predispose to SCD (e.g., anomalous coronary arteries) have no distinctive features on physical examination, and the presenting symptom may be an episode of SCD. Even underlying CAD that is not clinically apparent by history can lead to sudden cardiac death since acute changes in a nonobstructive plaque, such as rupture with thrombus formation, may result in a lethal arrhythmia followed by death.

Despite the limited ability of the patient history and physical examination to identify persons at high risk for SCD, it is important that all persons currently involved in or contemplating participating in athletic activities undergo baseline and periodic assessments. The preparticipation examination should ideally be performed approximately 6 weeks prior to training (to allow for rehabilitation and correction of problems). It is designed to detect conditions that may limit or exclude competition in certain sports, to identify preexisting conditions that might lead to injury, and to meet legal and insurance requirements.[12]

Patient History

Both the medical and family history of an athlete are crucial parts of the preparticipation examination. Zehender et al.[13] reviewed 146 cases of SCD reported in 12 studies and found that symptoms suggestive of a cardiac abnormality were present in one-third. Exercise-induced syncope is a particularly ominous finding since it can be suggestive of HCM, a serious conduction or heart rhythm abnormality, or valvular heart disease. Exertional chest pain can be due to myocardial ischemia, HCM, or aortic stenosis. Palpitations are often benign in athletes unless they are associated with syncope or presyncope. Extreme dyspnea or fatigue with exercise also requires a full evaluation, often in consultation with a cardiologist.

The following questions are helpful in obtaining a complete history pertaining to athletes and are taken from the *Preparticipation Physical Evaluation* monograph[14]:

1. Have you ever passed out during or after exercise?
2. Have you ever been dizzy during or after exercise?
3. Have you ever had chest pain during or after exercise?
4. Do you tire more quickly than your friends during exercise?
5. Have you ever had high blood pressure?
6. Have you ever been told that you have a heart murmur?
7. Have you ever had racing of your heart or skipped heartbeats?
8. Has anyone in your family died of heart problems or SCD before age 50?
9. Have you had a recent viral infection?
10. Do you currently or have you recently used any drugs (i.e., anabolic steroids, cocaine)?
11. Has a physician ever denied your participation in sports for a cardiac reason?

Middle-aged athletes who desire to begin a rigorous exercise program should be questioned carefully about their motives. It is not unusual to see people in this age group embark on an exercise program prompted by symptoms of ischemia.[15] The preparticipation physical exam allows the physician an opportunity to educate the older athlete regarding the symptoms of cardiac ischemia and the need for prompt medical attention. In a series of 18 exercise-related deaths reviewed by Thompson et al.,[16] up to 50% of the victims of SCD reported symptoms suggestive of cardiac ischemia to relatives but did not seek medical advice.

A family history of SCD at a young age should lead the examiner to consider the diagnosis of HCM, congenital coronary anomalies, atherosclerotic CAD, Marfan's syndrome, and congenital conduction system abnormalities such as the prolonged QT syndrome.

General Physical Examination

The setting for the preparticipation physical examination should be quiet and private and should allow the examiner to perform a careful evaluation, rather than a brief examination done in an assembly-line fashion. An outline of the general physical examination can be found in the comprehensive review by Smith et al.[12] Measurement of height and weight with comparison to standard charts is an excellent way to begin counseling individuals about eating disorders, diet, and weight control. Visual acuity can be assessed by a Snellen eye chart, and vision should be correctable to better than 20/200 (the legal blindness threshold). Myopia is commonly found in individuals with Marfan syndrome and may not be readily apparent since many athletes wear contact lenses.

Other systemic manifestations of Marfan syndrome include the following abnormalities[17]:

1. *Musculoskeletal system*: kyphoscoliosis, long limbs, long fingers and toes, joint hyperextensibility, chest-wall deformities, and high arched palate.
2. *Cardiovascular system*: aortic dilatation and/or insufficiency, aortic dissection, mitral valve prolapse and/or regurgitation, and aneurysms.
3. *Ocular system*: ectopic lens, myopia, and retinal detachment.
4. *Integumentary system*: striae and hernias.
5. *Neurologic system*: dural ectasia, learning disability, and myopathy.
6. *Pulmonary system*: apical pulmonary blebs and spontaneous pneumothorax.

Several simple assessments can be made during the physical examination which can identify musculoskeletal abnormalities that are consistent with Marfan syndrome. First, long limbs can be objectively assessed by measuring armspan width, upper body height (from the pubic symphysis to the top of the head), and lower body height (from the pubic symphysis down), as shown in Figure 4-1. Normally, height exceeds armspan width, but in Marfan syndrome the opposite is often true. Long fingers can be assessed by use of the wrist sign and the thumb sign (see Figures 4-2 and 4-3).

For practical purposes, the diagnosis of Marfan syndrome should be considered if the following criteria are met, as proposed by Pyeritz[19]:

1. The patient has a first-degree relative with Marfan syndrome and abnormalities in at least two of the systems listed above.
2. The patient does not have a family history of Marfan syndrome, but does have at least one musculoskeletal abnormality and abnormalities in at least two of the other systems mentioned above.

In the future, generic mapping may be available to help identify those persons with genetic evidence of Marfan syndrome.[20] Further recommendations for testing and exercise clearance of patients with Marfan syndrome are discussed further in Chapters 5 and 6.

Blood pressure should be measured with an appropriately sized cuff and in both arms. Coarctation of the aorta should be suspected if pressures in the right and left arms differ by more than 15–20 mm Hg. Blood pressures of the lower extremities can also be measured and are of particular importance for two patient groups: (1) younger persons suspected of having coarctation of the aorta and (2) older persons suspected of having peripheral arterial occlusive disease. Leg blood pressures can be measured in one of two ways: (1) apply a leg cuff at the lower thigh and listen with a stethoscope over the popliteal artery or (2) apply an arm cuff just above

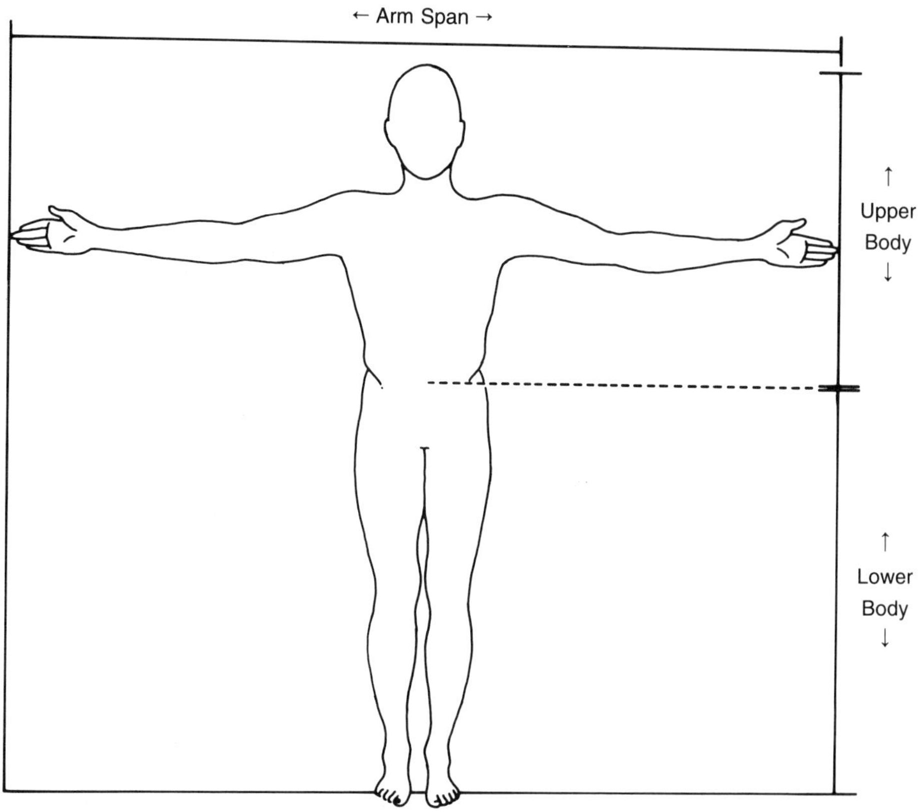

FIGURE 4-1. Assessment of long limbs in screening for Marfan syndrome: Normally, height exceeds armspan, but in Marfan syndrome armspan often exceeds height. The upper:lower body ratio is normally 0.92 ± 0.04 in white adults and 0.85 ± 0.03 in black adults. In Marfan syndrome, this ratio is typically less than these values.

the ankle at the level of the malleoli and listen to the posterior tibial or anterior tibial artery with a Doppler stethoscope. Normally, systolic blood pressures in the lower extremities are 5–15 mm Hg higher than in the upper extremities. When blood pressure is more than 20 mm Hg higher in the lower than in the upper extremities, significant aortic regurgitation should be suspected. When blood pressure in the lower extremities is less than that in the upper extremities, peripheral arterial occlusive disease or coarctation of the aorta should be suspected. Simultaneous palpation of the radial and femoral pulses is another excellent screening test for coarctation of the aorta (the femoral pulse will be delayed relative to the radial pulse in persons with coarctation of the aorta).

Resting hypertension need not prohibit a person from engaging in a regular exercise program or from exercise testing. As described in Chapter 7, patients with controlled, mild to moderate hypertension can be cleared for sports participation. Static exercise should be avoided in persons with severe or hard-to-control hyper-

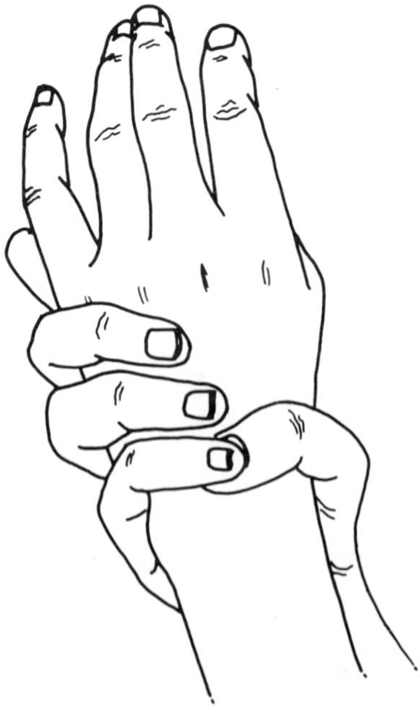

FIGURE 4-2. The wrist sign can be checked to identify persons with long fingers, consistent with Marfan syndrome. The patient grasps the left wrist just above the styloid process, using the right hand, and touches the thumb to the little finger of the right hand. A positive wrist sign occurs when the thumb and little finger overlap.

tension.[21] Exercise testing should be postponed if blood pressure is in excess of 200/120 mm Hg.[22]

The pulmonary and abdominal exams are performed just as in any general physical examination. Emphasis should be given to the clarity of lung sounds, the presence of wheezing or rubs, and the symmetry of chest excursion. The abdominal exam should be done in the supine position, with attention to the presence of

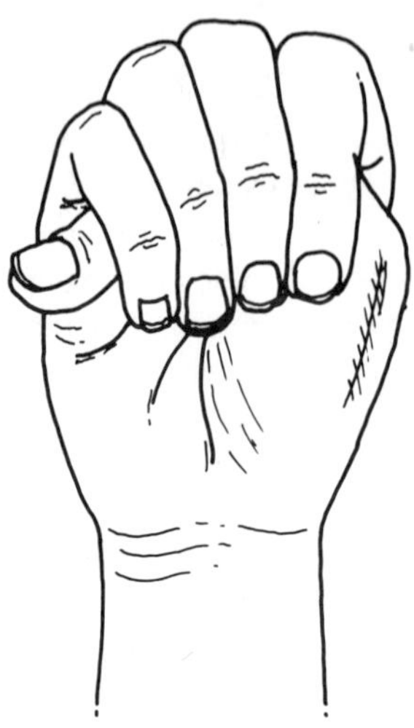

FIGURE 4-3. Long fingers can also be assessed by use of the thumb sign. The patient makes a fist with the thumb folded under the fingers. A positive thumb sign occurs when the tip of the thumb protudes beyond the little finger.

masses, palpation and estimation of the diameter of the abdominal aorta, and palpation of the liver and spleen.

The skin should be examined carefully for the presence of rashes such as impetigo, herpes, scabies, fungal infections, and molluscum contagiosum.[12] Any suspicious nevus or mass should be referred to a qualified dermatologist.

The genitourinary examination can be part of the preparticipation physical examination, but usually in men rather than in women. In males, testicular presence or absence, undescended testicles or masses, and inguinal hernias should be the focus of the exam.[12] Athletes should be advised to perform testicular self-examination on a regular basis. The female genitourinary examination can be performed depending on the expertise of the physician and the facilities available. In any case, a thorough menstrual history is essential, as is encouragement of the female athlete to have regular breast and pelvic examinations by a physician.

Cardiovascular Physical Examination

The cardiovascular examination should focus on identifying abnormal heart sounds and murmurs that may indicate a high-risk condition predisposing to sudden cardiac death, as described earlier in this chapter. Cardiac auscultation should be performed in both the supine and sitting positions. The first (S_1) and second (S_2) heart sounds should be evaluated for intensity and splitting. Splitting of S_1 can sometimes be detected with auscultation along the left sternal border due to mitral valve closure prior to tricuspid valve closure. This is a normal finding.[23] S_2 is usually single on expiration and split on inspiration. This is best heard along the left upper sternal border with the athlete sitting or standing. Fixed splitting of S_2 due to delayed pulmonic valve closure may indicate right bundle-branch block, pulmonic stenosis, or atrial septal defect.[23] Extra sounds on systole can sometimes be heard in patients with mitral valve prolapse (systolic click) and mitral stenosis (opening snap). Diastolic sounds, such as a soft S_3 or S_4 gallop, can often be heard in highly trained athletes.[24]

An important distinction in athletes, particularly young persons, is the difference between innocent and pathologic murmurs. Innocent murmurs are always systolic and decrease in intensity when the athlete changes from a supine to an upright position or during Valsalva's maneuver. They generally do not change with squatting. Diastolic murmurs should be considered pathologic in origin and require further evaluation. Other characteristics of innocent murmurs include short duration (i.e., not holosystolic), faint intensity, and no association with fixed splitting of S_2.[25] Table 4-2 presents the important differentiating points when distinguishing innocent systolic murmurs from the various types of pathologic murmurs.

While young patients may have innocent systolic murmurs, systolic murmurs in older patients (>50 years) may also be considered innocent in that they can be due to mild thickening or calcification of the aortic valve, a condition thought to occur as part of the aging process. Unlike significant aortic stenosis, innocent aortic "sclerosis" murmurs rarely radiate to the carotid, and the carotid upstroke is not diminished.

Positional changes (from supine to standing and from standing to squatting) and

TABLE 4-2. Characteristic changes in systolic murmurs during positional changes and Valsalva's manuever

	Supine to Standing	Standing to Squatting	Valsalva's Manuever
Innocent murmurs	Decreases	No change	No change
Aortic stenosis	Decreases	Increases	Decreases
Ventricular septal defect	Decreases or no change	Increases	Decreases
Mitral regurgitation	Decreases	Increases	Decreases
Hypertrophic cardiomyopathy	Increases	Decreases	Increases
Mitral valve prolapse	Increases	Decreases	Increases

Valsalva's maneuver can help distinguish between the various pathologic systolic murmurs that can be seen in the patient-athlete. As seen in Table 4-2, moving from the supine to the standing position or during the strain phase of Valsalva's maneuver generally *decreases* the intensity of most systolic murmurs, with two exceptions (in which case standing increases the murmur): (1) the murmur of HCM and (2) the late systolic murmur sometimes associated with mitral valve prolapse (MVP). Conversely, squatting will *increase* most pathologic systolic murmurs, with the same two exceptions (HCM and MVP), in which case squatting decreases the murmur.

Musculoskeletal Physical Examination

The complexity of the musculoskeletal examination varies depending on the expertise of the examiner. Extensive evaluation of certain joints (e.g., knee, shoulder) is indicated by a history of injury or a current problem and often involves referral to an orthopedist familiar with the care of athletes. A complete musculoskeletal examination is outlined in the review by Smith et al.,[12] and a shorter, 2-min screening examination can be found in the article by Dyment.[26] Participation in an exercise program should be deferred until any injuries identified on physical examination are rehabilitated.

SUMMARY

1. Exercise-related cardiac events are rare, limiting the application of extensive cardiovascular testing as part of a preparticipation evaluation. Furthermore, many persons who present with SCD were previously asymptomatic, making it impossible to identify all those at risk.
2. A thorough history aimed at detecting symptoms suggestive of underlying structural and atherosclerotic heart disease in combination with a physical examination focused on the common causes of sudden cardiovascular death can help the physician identify those few patient-athletes who are potentially at increased risk for SCD. Once identified, these patients should undergo further diagnostic

evaluation to help determine their eligibility for participation in a regular exercise program.

Acknowledgment

The author gratefully acknowledges the assistance of Ann Marie Belair in the preparation of this manuscript.

REFERENCES

1. Thompson PD, Funk EJ, Carlton RA, et al: Incidence of death during jogging in Rhode Island from 1975 through 1980. *JAMA* 247:2535–2538, 1982.
2. Siscovick DS, Weiss NS, Fletcher RH, et al: The incidence of primary cardiac arrest during vigorous exercise. *N Engl J Med* 311:874–877, 1984.
3. Haskell WL: Cardiovascular complications during exercise training of cardiac patients. *Circulation* 57:920–924, 1978.
4. Van Camp SP, Peterson RA: Cardiovascular complications of outpatient cardiac rehabilitation programs. *JAMA* 256:1160–1163, 1986.
5. Phillips M, Robinowitz M, Higgins JR, et al: Sudden cardiac death in Air Force recruits. *JAMA* 256:2696–2699, 1986.
6. Ragosta M, Crabtree J, Sturner WQ, et al: Death during recreational exercise in the State of Rhode Island. *Med Sci Sports Exerc* 16:339–342, 1984.
7. Maron BJ, Epstein SE, Roberts WC: Causes of sudden death in competitive athletes. *J Am Coll Cardiol* 7:204–214, 1986.
8. Virmani R, Roberts WC: Sudden cardiac death. *Hum Pathol* 18:485–492, 1987.
9. Maron BJ, Roberts WC, McAllister HA, et al: Sudden death in young athletes. *Circulation* 62:218–229, 1980.
10. Waller BF: Exercise-related sudden death in young (age ≤30 years) and old (age ≤30 years) conditioned subjects. *Cardiovasc Clin* 15:9–73, 1985.
11. Virmani R, Chun PKC, Goldstein RE, et al: Acute takeoffs of the coronary arteries along the aortic wall and congenital coronary ostial valve–like ridges: Association with sudden death. *J Am Coll Cardiol* 3:766–771, 1984.
12. Smith DM, Lombardo JA, Robinson JB: The preparticipation evaluation. *Primary Care* 18:777–807, 1991.
13. Zehender M, Meinertz T, Keul J, et al: ECG variants and cardiac arrhythmias in athletes: Clinical relevance and prognostic importance. *Am Heart J* 119:1378–1391, 1990.
14. Lombardo J, Nelson M, Smith D: *Preparticipation physical evaluation (PPE).* A joint publication: American Academy of Family Physicians, American Academy of Pediatrics, American Medical Society for Sports Medicine, American Orthopaedic Society for Sports Medicine, American Osteopathic Academy of Sports Medicine, 1992.
15. Fahrenbach MC, Thompson PD: The preparticipation sports examination. Cardiovascular considerations for screening. *Cardiol Clin* 10:319–328, 1992.
16. Thompson PD, Stern MP, Williams P, et al: Death during jogging or running: A study of 18 cases. *JAMA* 242:1265–1267, 1979.
17. Mellion MB: Diagnosing Marfan syndrome. *Heart Disease Stroke* 3:241–245, 1994.
18. Cantwell JD: Marfan's syndrome: Detection and management. *Physician Sportsmed* 14:51–55, 1986.
19. Pyeritz RE: The Marfan syndrome. *Am Fam Physician* 34:83–94, 1986.

20. Beighton P, de Paepe A, Hall JG, et al: Molecular nosology of heritable disorders of connective tissue. *Am J Med Genet* 42:431–438, 1992.
21. Maron BJ, Mitchell JH: 26th Bethesda Conference: Recommendations for determining eligibility for competition in athletes with cardiovascular abnormalities. *J Am Coll Cardiol* 24:845–899, 1994.
22. American College of Sports Medicine: *Guidelines for Exercise Testing and Exercise Prescription*, ed 3. Philadelphia, Lea and Febiger, 1986.
23. Rich BSE: Sudden death screening. *Med Clin North Am* 78:267–288, 1994.
24. Salem DN, Isner JM: Cardiac screening for athletes. *Orthop Clin North Am* 11:687–695, 1980.
25. Harvey WP, Knowlan DM: Techniques of clinical cardiovascular evaluation, with special emphasis of examination of athletes. In Waller BF, Harvey WP (eds): *Cardiovascular Evaluation of Athletes. Toward Recognizing Young Athletes at Risk of Sudden Death*. Newton, NJ, Laennec Publishing, 1993, p 31.
26. Dyment PG: The orthopedic component of the preparticipation examination. *Pediatr Ann* 21:157–162, 1992.

♦ CHAPTER FIVE ♦

SPECIAL PREPARTICIPATION TESTING

Todd D. Miller, M.D.

CASE EXAMPLE

A local high school district superintendent contacts you and asks you to help devise a preparticipation screening program for the members of the high school athletic teams in his district. One of the local football players died during a game in the previous season and was found on autopsy to have had hypertrophic cardiomyopathy (HCM). Since the regular preseason physical exam hadn't identified this condition, the superintendent asks you to devise a screening program that will utilize more advanced screening tools, such as electrocardiography, chest x-rays, and echocardiography to prevent sudden deaths in the future. What is your advice to the superintendent? Would your advice be different if you were asked to develop a screening procedure for older athletes? What testing would be appropriate for patient-athletes with preexisting cardiovascular disease?

INTRODUCTION

Exercise-related sudden death occurs in two general groups of people. These deaths are particularly shocking when they occur in a presumably healthy young person, especially a competitive athlete. Even when a patient with known cardiovascular disease dies suddenly during exercise, this event generally is unexpected because the patient usually has been doing well clinically. Exercise-related deaths focus attention on current methods of preparticipation evaluation of individuals before engaging in exercise programs. The common assumption is that better methods of preparticipation testing and counseling might prevent some of these deaths.

SPECIAL PREPARTICIPATION TESTING IN PERSONS AT HIGH RISK FOR CARDIOVASCULAR DISEASES

Exercise-related deaths generate considerable interest in the news media, as demonstrated by the coverage of such high-profile individuals as Jim Fixx (runner), Reggie Lewis (Boston Celtics basketball player), and Hank Gathers (Loyola Marymount University basketball player). However, these events are very rare. Estimates of occurrence range from 1 death per year among every 250,000 young athletes[1] to 1 death annually among every 5000 to 20,000 older exercisers.[2–5] The goal of preparticipation screening is to identify individuals at high risk of these very uncommon events. However, in view of the rare occurrence of these events, even high-risk individuals relative to the general population have a very low absolute risk of dying.

Most athletes with exercise-related death are found to have an identifiable structural cardiovascular abnormality at postmortem examination. While there is no direct proof that these conditions cause sudden death during exercise (mechanisms have not been proven), it is generally accepted that they are responsible for sudden death, most likely by predisposing some individuals who have these conditions to a fatal arrhythmia. Less commonly, primary arrhythmias may occur in individuals without structural heart disease.

Table 5-1 lists cardiovascular abnormalities that have been associated or potentially could be associated with sudden death during exercise. This subject has been reviewed previously by Waller,[6] as described in Chapter 4. An attractive approach to preparticipation screening of patient-athletes is to review the conditions that have been associated with exercise-related death and then to examine current methods of detecting these conditions in asymptomatic individuals. Since the prevalence of these conditions varies by age, the conditions in younger and older exercisers are considered in detail below.

Conditions Associated with Exercise-Related Deaths in Athletes Younger Than Age 30

The two most common conditions associated with exercise-related deaths in young athletes are congenital coronary anomalies[6] and HCM.[7,8] These two condi-

TABLE 5-1. Cardiovascular conditions associated or potentially associated with exercise-related death

Coronary Arteries
- Atherosclerosis
- Congenital anomalies (primarily anomalous origins)
- Spasm
- Myocardial bridging (tunneled epicardial coronary artery)
- Nonatherosclerotic narrowing of the atrioventricular node artery
- Kawasaki's disease (coronary arteries)
- Dissection

Myocardium
- Hypertrophic cardiomyopathy
- Idiopathic dilated cardiomyopathy
- Myocarditis
- Arrhythmogenic right ventricular dysplasia

Cardiac Valves
- Mitral valve prolapse (floppy mitral valve)
- Aortic stenosis—congenital or acquired
- Other congenital heart lesions—tetralogy of Fallot, Ebstein's anomaly, pulmonary vascular obstruction

Aorta
- Dissection (with or without Marfan syndrome)

Primary arrhythmias
- Wolff-Parkinson-White syndrome
- Long QT syndrome
- Idiopathic exercise-induced ventricular tachycardia

Environmental agents
- Antiarrhythmic medications
- Cardiovascular toxins (e.g., cocaine)

tions combined account for 60–70% of the structural cardiovascular abnormalities found at postmortem exam in this younger population. Most congenital coronary anomalies include anomalous origin of the coronary arteries, the most common of which is origin of the left main coronary artery from the right sinus of Valsalva, with passage between the aorta and the pulmonary trunk. Other anomalies include a single epicardial coronary artery and hypoplastic epicardial coronary arteries. HCM includes classic asymmetric septal hypertrophy with outflow obstruction and concentric left ventricular hypertrophy.

Conditions other than congenital coronary anomalies and HCM are very uncommon. Other structural abnormalities of the coronary arteries include atherosclerotic disease, nonatherosclerotic narrowing of the atrioventricular node artery, Kawasaki's disease, and myocardial bridging.[6,9–12] Significant atherosclerotic coronary artery disease is uncommon in this age group but has been associated with about 5% of exercise-related deaths.[6] Nonatherosclerotic narrowing (fibromuscular dysplasia) of the coronary arteries occurs and involves the atrioventricular node branch.[11] Kawasaki's disease, or coronary arteritis, results in aneurysmal dilatation and in situ thrombosis in the coronary arteries.[10] *Myocardial bridging* is the term applied to tunneling of a portion of an epicardial coronary artery, usually the left anterior descending artery, through the myocardium.[9,12] Other conditions affecting the coronary arteries include exercise-induced coronary arterial spasm and spontaneous coronary arterial dissection.[6]

Conditions affecting the myocardium other than HCM include idiopathic dilated cardiomyopathy and myocarditis.[6–8,10] A unique form of cardiomyopathy is arrhythmogenic right ventricular dysplasia.[13] This disorder typically involves the right ventricle, with no or little left ventricular involvement. The hallmark of the diagnosis is histologic demonstration of fat or fat and fibrous tissue replacing right ventricular myocardium. Morphologically, there is usually enlargement and reduction in function of the right ventricle.[13] Clinically, these patients often present with nonsustained or sustained ventricular tachycardia with left bundle branch block morphology.[14] Although rarely reported in other series, this entity was found in nearly 30% of young athletes dying suddenly in a region of northern Italy.[15,16]

A few remaining structural cardiovascular abnormalities have been associated with sudden death in the young athlete. Mitral valve prolapse has been the most commonly reported valvular heart disease.[6] Severe aortic stenosis is a potential cause of sudden death during exercise. Dissection or rupture of the ascending aorta, either in individuals with Marfan syndrome or as an isolated entity, has also occurred.[6]

A variety of atrial and ventricular arrhythmias have been reported in athletes.[17] Most of these arrhythmias are benign. Even the majority of young adults with exercise-induced ventricular tachycardia who have a structurally normal heart generally have a good prognosis.[18] However, life-threatening arrhythmias do occur in a small percentage of athletes.[19] Occasionally, these arrhythmias are markers of occult cardiomyopathy or myocarditis. The prevalence of life-threatening arrhythmias induced by exercise in individuals with underlying arrhythmogenic substrate, such as Wolff-Parkinson-White syndrome or long-QT interval syndrome, is not known. Athletes with these conditions have been reported to develop life-threatening arrhythmias.[19,20]

A number of therapeutic and nontherapeutic agents may predispose the athlete to sudden death. All of the antiarrhythmic medications carry a small risk of proarrhythmia.[21] Proarrhythmia is defined as a new arrhythmia or worsening of a preexisting arrhythmia after initiation of antiarrhythmic medication. These arrhythmias are often life-threatening ventricular arrhythmias, such as torsade de pointes. They may be unmasked only during exercise. Antiarrhythmic medications are the prototype of proarrhythmia drugs. A more legitimate concern is the use of nontherapeutic drugs by the athlete. Cocaine can cause a number of adverse cardiovascular effects, including coronary atherosclerosis, coronary artery spasm, cardiomyopathy, stroke, and cardiac arrhythmias.[22] It has been implicated in the premature deaths of athletes.

Conditions Associated with Exercise-Related Deaths in Patients Older Than Age 30

The disease entity found in almost all exercise-related deaths in adults over age 30 is atherosclerotic coronary artery disease.[4,6,23] In the review by Waller,[6] 97% of conditioned subjects over age 30 years studied at autopsy had atherosclerotic coronary artery disease. Although any of the entities listed in Table 5-1 theoretically could cause sudden death during exercise in adults over age 30, most of these conditions have never been reported in older exercisers at autopsy.

Challenges Posed by Screening the General Population

The formidable challenge for preparticipation screening is to identify the very rare individual at risk of experiencing sudden death during or shortly after exercise. From a practical standpoint, this means trying to identify the young athlete who has hypertrophic cardiomyopathy or a congenital coronary anomaly and the older exerciser who has atherosclerotic coronary artery disease. The prevalence of these conditions in the general population is very low. The prevalence of HCM is estimated to be 0.1% in adults aged 23 to 35 years.[24] The prevalence of congenital coronary artery anomalies in the general population is unknown. In a study of 1273 athletes ranging in age from 13 to 49 years who underwent echocardiography with technically satisfactory images, Pelliccia et al.[25] reported that 28 athletes had minor variants of coronary artery anatomy, but there were no instances of anomalous origin of the coronary arteries. In the Coronary Artery Surgery Study, which enrolled almost 25,000 primary symptomatic older adults with known or presumed coronary artery disease who underwent coronary angiography, the prevalence of coronary artery anomalies was 0.3%.[26] Only nine patients had anomalous origin of the left main artery, and in only one of these patients did the left main artery travel between the great vessels. Coronary artery disease is more prevalent in the older general population than are HCM and coronary anomalies in the younger population, but nonetheless it is still relatively uncommon. The average prevalence is about 4%, ranging from 0.3% in women aged 30–39 years to 12% in men aged 60–69 years.[27]

Using the History and Physical Examination to Guide Laboratory Testing

The cornerstone of any screening evaluation always consists of a focused history and a physical exam (see Chapter 4). When necessary, laboratory testing can be performed to evaluate the cardiovascular system more thoroughly. Table 5-2 lists available laboratory tests, categorized into three general groups on the basis of availability, expense, and safety. The important issue for preparticipation screening is to select individuals who might benefit from group I or Group II testing. In general, group III testing is performed only if there are significant abnormalities on the noninvasive laboratory studies or if clinical findings are highly suggestive of an underlying life-threatening abnormality and the results of other tests have been negative.

The role of the preparticipation history and physical examination has been thoroughly addressed in Chapter 4 and elsewhere.[28] However, some comments are warranted concerning the decision to proceed with laboratory testing based on findings detected on the screening history and physical examination.

TABLE 5-2. Laboratory tests available for further assessment of the cardiovascular system

Group I (widely available, least expensive, noninvasive)
Electrocardiogram
Chest x-ray
Group II (commonly available, moderate expensive, noninvasive)
Exercise testing
Echocardiography and other imaging modalities (CT scanning, magnetic resonance imaging)
Ambulatory electrocardiography
Tilt-table testing
Group III (restricted availability, most expensive, invasive)
Cardiac catheterization (including coronary angiography)
Endomyocardial biopsy
Electrophysiologic testing

The vast majority of individuals undergoing preparticipation screening are asymptomatic. Some athletes describe minor, infrequent, and atypical symptoms which usually do not need to be pursued further. However, for the rare individual who describes typical cardiac symptoms (angina, excessive exertional dyspnea, syncope, frequent palpitations) or a past history of cardiovascular disease, a more extensive evaluation is warranted. Specific testing will depend on the clinical situation. For instance, in the young athlete with a history of exercise-related syncope, treadmill testing to detect an exercise-related arrhythmia and echocardiography to exclude structural heart disease are usually performed. Since vasodepressor (neurocardiogenic) syncope is a common cause of syncope in this setting, tilt-table testing may be useful to confirm this diagnosis.[29] For the older exerciser with a history of angina, stress testing is appropriate.

Even if the participant is asymptomatic, elements of the family or social history may heighten concern about possible occult cardiovascular disease. In the young athlete, a family history of sudden death in a first-degree relative or other close relative at a young age (generally age 40 or younger) should raise the possibility of HCM, arrhythmogenic right ventricular dysplasia, or long QT syndrome. All of these entities occur sporadically but also are known to occur in families, with autosomal dominant transmission reported in at least some families.[30–35] Electrocardiography and echocardiography should usually be performed in individuals with a positive family history. A history of significant cocaine use increases the likelihood of developing structural heart disease and may prompt further evaluation.

In the older individual, the presence of cardiac risk factors is related to the likelihood of developing atherosclerotic coronary artery disease. Although the detection and treatment of risk factors does have a significant impact on the population as a whole from a public health standpoint, identification of risk factors in an individual usually has very modest prognostic value. For instance, in the Multiple Risk Factor Intervention Trial (MRFIT),[36] the presence of one of the traditional cardiac risk factors was associated with approximately a doubling of the risk of dying during the next 6 years of follow-up, but the absolute risk was 4 to 5 per 1000 individuals with the risk factor versus 2 per 1000 individuals without the risk factor.[36] A clinical concept that is not commonly appreciated is that the presence of risk factors, even multiple risk factors, has much weaker predictive value for identifying individuals with coronary artery disease than does the symptomatic status of the individual.[37,38]

The preparticipation physical examination is also normal in the vast majority of individuals, including not only those with normal cardiovascular systems but also the majority of those with coronary artery disease and congenital coronary anomalies and even those with HCM.[28] Any individual suspected of having HCM or significant underlying valvular heart disease on the basis of the physical examination (see Chapter 4) should be considered for echocardiography. Trained athletes can occasionally have soft systolic murmurs and third or fourth heart sounds.[39] The differentiation between these fairly commonly detected, benign, "innocent" physical findings and significant valvular pathology can usually be accomplished by careful physical examination, although echocardiography may occasionally be necessary in difficult cases.

Thus, although rare individuals have worrisome findings detected by the history or physical exam that warrant further evaluation, most individuals undergoing preparticipation evaluation have either a completely normal history and physical exam or only mild abnormalities that do not need to be pursued further. The issue then arises of whether laboratory testing should be performed routinely to detect individuals with underlying cardiovascular abnormalities associated with exercise-related death.

The Screening Electrocardiogram and Chest X-Ray

Group I tests may be abnormal in conditions associated with exercise-related death. Occasionally, these studies yield pathognomonic findings, such as a long QT internal in an individual with the long QT syndrome or a markedly widened mediastinum with left ventricular enlargement in an individual with aortic root enlargement with aortic insufficiency. At other times, these tests yield findings highly suggestive of an underlying disorder, such as left ventricular hypertrophy in an individual with hypertrophic cardiomyopathy or significant Q waves in an individual with an old, silent myocardial infarction. Very often, however, these studies are normal (low sensitivity) in many of the conditions associated with exercise-related death, or they demonstrate minor abnormalities seen in many conditions (low specificity). In particular, athletes frequently have electrocardiographic evidence of left or right ventricular hypertrophy and repolarization abnormalities, as well as chest x-ray evidence of cardiomegaly.[39] Group I tests have not come into routine use for preparticipation screening, largely due to their limited sensitivity and specificity. Although they are relatively inexpensive compared to other laboratory tests, their widespread use would add considerable cost to preparticipation screening. Since group I tests are ineffective for screening, the question arises of whether more sophisticated screening tests should be routinely utilized. From a practical standpoint, this would mean performing echocardiography on all young athletes and exercise treadmill testing on all older exercisers.

Screening Echocardiography in the Young Athlete

Theoretically, transthoracic echocardiography is a useful tool to detect the conditions associated with exercise-related death in the young athlete. Echocardiography is considered the gold standard for assessment of HCM and can detect anomalous origin of the coronary arteries.[40] It can also play a useful and/or definitive role in the assessment of most of the conditions listed in Table 5-1.

There are some potential limitations in using echocardiography to screen for these conditions. Its sensitivity for detecting many of these conditions is not known. Although classic HCM with asymmetric septal hypertrophy and left ventricular outflow tract obstruction likely would not be missed, variants of left ventricular hypertrophy, such as regional hypertrophy not involving the septum, could be missed. Another potential limitation involves the overlap that occurs between mild forms of cardiomyopathy and changes in left ventricular anatomy seen in "athletic heart syndrome."[39,41] Compared to controls, left ventricular end-diastolic diameter tends to be approximately 10% greater and left ventricular wall thickness 15–20% greater in athletes.[40,42] In general, athletes involved in isotonic (dynamic) sports tend to develop more chamber enlargement and less increase in wall thickness (eccentric hypertrophy), whereas those involved in isometric (static) sports tend to develop increased wall thickness with little change in cavity dimension (concentric hypertrophy).[39,41–43] In athletes with increased wall thickness, the distinction between increased thickness due to athletic training and true pathologic left ventricular hypertrophy can usually be made by Doppler assessment of diastolic filling, which is normal in athletes and abnormal in cardiomyopathy.[41,42,44] "Detraining" for a couple of weeks results in regression of a left ventricular mass[41] and can be useful in difficult cases. Athletic training has also been associated with an increased prevalence of mitral and tricuspid regurgitation measured by Doppler echocardiography.[45] An important caveat to remember when using echocardiography in an athletic population is that abnormal findings do not necessarily represent significant cardiac pathology.

Another issue to consider when using echocardiography to detect HCM is the age of the patient. In a series of 39 children with a family history or morphologic evidence of HCM, Maron et al.[46] described a marked increase in average left ventricular wall thickness ranging from 6 to 23 mm in 22 of these patients between the average ages of 11 and 16 years, including 5 patients who developed a morphologic change in the appearance of the heart from normal to hypertrophic. An echocardiogram later in life may be necessary to exclude HCM in an individual with a normal echocardiogram at a young age.

The value of screening large groups of young athletes with echocardiography to detect cardiovascular disease has been studied.[25,47,48] As noted earlier, Pelliccia et al.[25] reported that 28 of 1273 athletes with technically satisfactory echocardiographic images had coronary artery anomalies, but all of these anomalies were only minor variants and none of these individuals had anomalous origin of the left main or right coronary arteries. In a study of 501 intercollegiate athletes at the University of Maryland who underwent a screening history, physical examination, and electrocardiogram, 90 had abnormalities and were referred for echocardiography. None of these athletes had definite evidence of a cardiovascular condition associated with exercise-related death, although 14 had mild mitral valve prolapse and 3 had mild ventricular septal hypertrophy.[47] In another study of 265 primarily black collegiate athletes who underwent screening echocardiography, 11% had mitral valve prolapse, 11% had modestly increased septal thickness, and 1 had an atrial septal defect, but none had definite evidence of a disorder considered to be potentially life-threatening.[48]

Although screening echocardiography may appear to be a rational approach for detecting the athlete at high risk of exercise-related death, the above studies suggest that it is not clinically useful or cost effective for this purpose.

Screening Exercise Tests in the Older Exerciser

The goal of screening in the exerciser over 30 years of age is primarily to detect coronary artery disease. Before discussing screening exercise testing for the older exerciser, however, some issues relating to treatment of coronary artery disease and to screening exercise testing in the general population will be reviewed.

Coronary artery bypass surgery does improve survival in some patients with coronary artery disease. Prospective randomized trials have shown that individuals with left main artery and/or three-vessel disease, especially if associated with reduced left ventricular global function, have a survival advantage when treated initially with bypass surgery versus medication.[49–51] Although most of the patients in these studies were symptomatic, it is generally believed that the same advantage should apply to asymptomatic individuals. Most patients with only one- or two-vessel coronary artery disease are at relatively low risk for future cardiac death over the next several years, and bypass surgery generally has not been shown to enhance survival over medical therapy,[50,52] although selected patients may benefit.[53,54] Thus, bypass surgery improves survival in only a small percentage of patients. Additionally, bypass surgery has not been shown to lower the risk of future myocardial infarction compared to treatment with medical therapy.[52,53]

There is no study which shows that treatment with coronary angioplasty or anti-ischemic medication (except beta blockers after myocardial infarction) improves survival or reduces the risk of myocardial infarction in patients with coronary artery disease. A recent study did show a nonsignificant trend toward fewer adverse cardiac events in asymptomatic or minimally symptomatic patients treated with atenolol versus placebo.[55] The only medication that has been shown to be beneficial for the primary prevention of myocardial infarction is aspirin.[56]

One reason for not performing screening exercise testing in the general population is that there is very little evidence that any form of treatment can change the natural history of many patients with coronary artery disease. Another reason relates to the limitations of the test. In symptomatic individuals, in whom the prevalence of coronary artery disease is relatively high, exercise testing performs reasonably well, with average sensitivity of 65–70% and specificity of 75–80%.[57] However, in the asymptomatic population, the test is less accurate. Since the prevalence of disease in the general population is ≤5%,[27] most "positive" stress tests (approximately 80%) will be false positives.[58] The prognostic value of screening exercise testing in the general population is also poor. Studies using "hard" endpoints (cardiac death or nonfatal myocardial infarction) have reported that testing misses two-thirds of patients who have future events, and the predictive value of a positive test (the percentage of individuals with a positive test who subsequently experience a cardiac event) is only 5%.[59–61] The routine use of screening exercise testing in the general population is not recommended.[62]

Stress testing with nuclear or echocardiographic imaging enhances the accuracy of standard stress testing. However, the accuracy of the imaging procedures is also limited in the asymptomatic general population (due to the low prevalence of disease). These imaging techniques add considerable cost to the test and also are not routinely recommended. It is unknown whether newer screening techniques, such as computed tomography (CT) scanning for detection of coronary artery calcification,[63] will prove to be more useful than standard exercise testing.

The question arises of whether people who exercise regularly should be approached differently from nonexercisers for screening treadmill testing. Although regular physical activity is associated with an overall lower mortality risk,[64] there is a risk of sudden cardiac death during acute exercise that is on the order of 1 in approximately 500,000 hours of participation.[4,65,66] The obvious concern is that an asymptomatic person with underlying coronary artery disease could theoretically develop significant ischemia during exercise, which could precipitate cardiac arrest. Even if a person does not have left main or three-vessel coronary artery disease (the conditions for which bypass surgery has been associated with improved survival), knowledge of the presence of any underlying coronary disease in the exerciser might be useful in other ways. Medication could be initiated in an attempt to lessen the severity of exercise-induced ischemia, or the exercise prescription might be revised to keep the exercise heart rate below the ischemic threshold. Whether the implementation of these measures can actually reduce the risk of sudden death during exercise has never been proved, but these measures are often followed in clinical practice.

There are very little data addressing the specific issue of the ability of exercise testing to identify individuals who experience cardiac events during exercise. In the only published study on this subject, Siscovick et al.[67] reported results similar to those of earlier studies evaluating total, not just exercise-related, events. Subjects with a positive test were more likely to experience exercise-related myocardial infarction or cardiac death than those with a negative test, but sensitivity was only 18% and the predictive value of a positive test was a disappointing 4%.

Preparticipation screening exercise testing in the asymptomatic older individual is controversial. The Task Force on Exercise Testing for the American College of Cardiology and the American Heart Association considered screening exercise testing in sedentary men over age 40 who are beginning a vigorous exercise program a class II indication (a condition for which exercise testing is frequently used but in which there is a divergence of opinion with respect to value and appropriateness).[62] A more recent report from the American Heart Association recommended that individuals 40 years of age or older or with two or more major coronary risk factors should undergo a symptom-limited, maximum exercise test if they are planning to participate in vigorous exercise (such as jogging or running).[66] The

American College of Sports Medicine's previous recommendations were very similar, except that the age cutoffs were defined as 40 or older for men and 50 or older for women and vigorous exercise was defined as intensity >60% VO_2max.[68] A more recent recommendation, issued jointly by this organization and the Centers for Disease Control and Prevention, stated that these groups of individuals "should consult their physicians to design a safe, effective program."[69]

Guidelines for Preparticipation Screening Tests

Recommended guidelines for both the young athlete and the older exerciser are summarized in Table 5-3. Laboratory testing cannot be routinely recommended for the young athlete. Due to the extremely low prevalence of the entities associated with sudden death during exercise in this population, hundreds, if not thousands, of athletes would need to be screened to detect an individual with one of these conditions. Laboratory testing in this population should be based on the athlete's personal history of cardiac symptoms, positive family history, or abnormal findings on physical examination. Testing should include an electrocardiogram, echocardiogram, and, in selected individuals, a chest x-ray and other group II tests.[28] Laboratory testing in the older population should be performed in any individual with symptoms typical of heart disease. An electrocardiogram and an exercise treadmill test are the initial procedures performed in individuals with symptoms consistent with ischemic heart disease. Additional testing may be warranted based on other features of the history or findings on physical exam. The role of screening exercise testing in the asymptomatic older individual remains controversial. Despite the very modest predictive value of cardiac risk factors in the individual and the lack of data indicating that screening exercise testing can accurately identify individuals at risk for an exercise-related cardiac event, both the American Heart Association[66] and the American College of Sports Medicine[68] recommended exercise testing in individuals

TABLE 5-3. Conditions in which preparticipation laboratory testing is recommended

In the younger athlete*
- Personal history of angina, congestive heart failure, or syncope
- Family history of HCM, arrhythmogenic right ventricular dysplasia, long QT syndrome, or sudden death in a first-degree relative aged 40 or younger
- Findings on physical examination suggesting HCM or clinically significant valvular disease

In the older athlete*
- Personal history of angina or other cardiac symptoms
- Age 40 or older and planning a vigorous exercise program†
- Two or more coronary risk factors and planning a vigorous exercise program†

*In the younger athlete, testing usually consists of an electrocardiogram and an echocardiogram and, in the older athlete, an electrocardiogram and a stress test, although other testing may be performed in selected circumstances.

†Stress testing for these indications is controversial but is recommended by the American Heart Association[68] and the American College of Sports Medicine.[69]

who either are 40 years of age or older or who have two or more risk factors for coronary artery disease and plan to exercise vigorously. The clinician should be aware of the limitations of testing in this situation. A positive test leads to the dilemma of trying to resolve true-positive from false-positive results, which often leads to further testing with nuclear or echocardiographic imaging and sometimes coronary angiography. This approach is expensive, and the practice of preparticipation exercise testing is likely to be scrutinized even more closely as we move into an era of increasing financial constraints.

SPECIAL PREPARTICIPATION TESTING IN PERSONS WITH PREEXISTING CARDIOVASCULAR DISEASES

This section applies to the noncompetitive or recreational athlete with established cardiovascular disease and addresses individuals who are exercising primarily for fitness purposes. The reader who is interested in guidelines for the competitive athlete is referred to the comprehensive publication produced at the 26th Bethesda Conference by the American College of Cardiology and the American College of Sports Medicine.[70]

Some form of exercise is likely to be valuable for all individuals, regardless of their underlying cardiovascular disease. As noted earlier, there does appear to be a short-term risk of sudden death associated with acute exercise,[4,65,66] but this risk needs to be weighed against the larger long-term risk of a sedentary lifestyle.[64,69] The goal of the exercise prescription for the individual with known cardiovascular disease is to provide a program that not only is beneficial from a conditioning standpoint but also is as safe as possible.

There will always be some uncertainty and imprecision when attempting to judge an individual patient's risk of death during exercise. Part of this uncertainty relates to the fact that the cause of exercise-related death is not completely understood. The conditions listed in Table 5-1 have only been associated with sudden death during or after exercise and, in fact, may not be causal. For instance, conditions such as mitral valve prolapse or myocardial bridging have been reported to exist in 5–10% of the general population but have been found in only a few people who have died suddenly during exercise. It is extremely unlikely that individuals with either of these conditions will die suddenly during exercise. Even in individuals with conditions that are uncommon and appear more likely to be the cause of sudden death, the mechanism remains unknown. Some individuals with HCM die during minimal activity, whereas other individuals compete in high-intensity sports for years without incident.[71] This point is perhaps best illustrated by the case of Pete Maravich, who had a single coronary artery and died at age 40. He successfully completed a professional basketball career without incident and yet died after retiring from professional sports during an informal basketball game.

The limitations of the exercise test for screening purposes were addressed earlier. The exercise test is more useful for formulating an exercise prescription for patients with known coronary artery disease. The simple presence or absence of ST segment depression, the variable that is most important for diagnostic testing, is of little value in patients with established disease. Much more useful is the ascertainment of the exercise intensity at which angina and/or ST segment depression (the ischemic threshold) occur. In patients with coronary artery disease as well as those with other cardiovascular diseases, assessment of the blood pressure response to exercise and assessment of arrhythmias can also be useful when formulating the exercise prescription.

Exercise Testing to Guide Exercise Prescription in Patients with Established Coronary Artery Disease

In general, patients with coronary artery disease should undergo exercise treadmill or cycle ergometer testing before beginning a program of exercise training. It has never been proved that exercising above the ischemic threshold is harmful, but there are anecdotal reports of individuals with known coronary artery disease performing excessive levels of exercise who experienced adverse events.[6,72] It is common practice to recommend that the intensity of exercise be kept below the ischemic threshold. This can be accomplished by teaching the individual pulse monitoring and advising that the exercise heart rate be maintained 10 beats per minute or more below the ischemic threshold (see Chapter 7). In the individual with exercise-induced angina, the ischemic threshold can be determined by the onset of either angina or 1.0 mm of ST segment depression, whichever comes first. In the individual with silent exercise ischemia, the anginal threshold is determined by the onset of 1.0 mm ST segment depression.

Although exercise training formerly was proscribed for patients with congestive heart failure, currently it is believed to be beneficial for most of these patients.[73,74] An exercise test can be especially helpful for these patients prior to beginning an exercise program. In addition to determining the ischemic threshold, particular attention should be paid to the development of excessive exertional dyspnea, as well as the development of arrhythmias. Since some individuals with reduced left ventricular systolic function become anaerobic very early in exercise, cardiopulmonary exercise testing can be used to determine the anaerobic threshold in these patients. However, the value of basing the exercise prescription on the anaerobic threshold for patients with congestive heart failure has yet to be demonstrated.

Exercise testing should certainly be performed in patients with coronary artery disease who are taking antiarrhythmic agents, especially those who have reduced left ventricular systolic function and a history of ventricular arrhythmias and/or sudden death. A small percentage of patients taking antiarrhythmic medications will experience a proarrhythmic effect.[21] Occasionally, this effect may be unmasked only during exercise.

The preparticipation exercise test should try to simulate as closely as possible the primary activity that the patient pursues. The majority of patients with coronary artery disease participate in walking/jogging or cycling programs. In these individuals, an exercise test that simulates their aerobic exercise program is appropriate, such as a treadmill or cycle ergometer test. Some individuals swim as their main mode of exercise. Since most exercise laboratories cannot perform a swimming exercise test, individuals interested in swimming usually undergo a treadmill or cycle ergometer test to determine the ischemic threshold. The same applies to patients who play racquet sports. Although weight lifting was once believed to be detrimental for patients with coronary artery disease, moderate weight lifting has been shown to be safe for carefully selected individuals.[75] Monitoring of vital signs and an electrocardiogram can be performed in the exercise laboratory during lifting to evaluate the safety of this activity.

The necessity of repeat testing for patients with coronary artery disease involved in an exercise program is not known. Since coronary artery disease is a progressive process, the rationale for repeat testing is to determine if the ischemic threshold is changing over time, which might necessitate further diagnostic testing or require altering the exercise prescription. Certainly, repeat testing should be performed after a significant clinical event (e.g., myocardial infarction). However, the value of testing at annual or other intervals in individuals who are doing well clinically has not been studied.

Testing to Guide Exercise Prescription in Patients with Cardiovascular Disorders Other Than Coronary Artery Disease

There are very little published data on the value of testing before formulating an exercise prescription in patients with cardiovascular disorders other than coronary artery disease. Since this group of patients has known disease, some type of testing likely has been done in the past and does not need to be repeated prior to beginning an exercise program simply to confirm the diagnosis. However, there are selected situations in which exercise testing may be helpful.

In patients with disorders that may affect coronary blood flow, such as anomalous coronary arteries, Kawasaki's disease, myocardial bridging, and coronary artery spasm, exercise testing may be helpful to determine the ischemic threshold, just as it is used in patients with atherosclerotic coronary artery disease. Since these disorders generally are not progressive, serial testing should not be necessary unless there has been a significant change in clinical status (e.g., after a change in medication in a patient with coronary artery spasm or following surgery to reimplant the coronary arteries in a patient with anomalous coronary arteries).

Exercise testing may occasionally be helpful in patients with other cardiovascular disorders not involving the coronary arteries, primarily to monitor symptoms, the hemodynamic (blood pressure) response to exercise, and the cardiac rhythm. These disorders include HCM, moderate or moderately severe aortic stenosis, idiopathic dilated cardiomyopathy, right ventricular dysplasia, pulmonary hypertension, and the occasional patient with poorly controlled systemic hypertension. Although several of these disorders are often considered contraindications to maximal exercise testing, cautious submaximal testing to a level of exercise that matches the intensity at which the individual will be performing on a regular basis can be helpful for assessing the safety of the exercise program.[66] Testing of these patients is generally performed under the supervision of a cardiologist. Particular attention is paid to symptoms of presyncope or excessive dyspnea, the blood pressure response to exercise, and the development of arrhythmia. The ST segment response in this setting is often nonspecific and is not useful for guiding further testing or for formulating the exercise prescription. The target heart rate for the exercise prescription should be 10 beats per minute or more below the heart rate at which any ominous symptoms or signs develop.

Individuals with certain cardiovascular conditions that progress over time will need periodic clinical, and at times echocardiographic, assessment to monitor for progression of disease. These conditions include aortic stenosis for assessment of a progressively increasing valve gradient, mitral valve prolapse with severe mitral regurgitation for assessment of deterioration in left ventricular function, and Marfan syndrome for assessment of an enlarging aortic root. Surgery is usually performed for these conditions when certain thresholds are met. Whether patients with these conditions who exercise regularly should undergo more frequent assessment compared to sedentary individuals is not known.

Guidelines for Preparticipation Testing in Patients with Preexisting Cardiovascular Disease

Exercise testing is useful in patients with coronary artery disease for determining the ischemic threshold. Exercise testing may also be helpful in patients with coronary artery disease or other selected cardiovascular conditions to assess the risk of developing an adverse hemodynamic response or arrhythmia during exercise.

SUMMARY

1. Because it is rare to find high-risk athletes in the general population, extensive testing is generally not indicated to screen the general population prior to initiating an exercise program.
2. Persons identified by their history or physical examination as being at high risk for dangerous cardiovascular disorders often require extensive preparticipation testing, such as electrocardiography, echocardiography, exercise testing, nuclear imaging studies, or even angiography (see Chapter 6 and 7). The yield of such testing is generally greatest in patients who either are symptomatic or who have a strong family history of cardiovascular disease.
3. Preparticipation exercise testing is of particular importance in patients with preexisting cardiovascular disorders since it provides not only prognostic and diagnostic information but also information regarding the intensity threshold under which the patient-athlete can safely exercise without becoming symptomatic (having significant ischemia, angina, hypotension, or dysrhythmias, for example).

REFERENCES

1. Ades PA: Preventing sudden death. Cardiovascular screening of young athletes. *Phys Sportsmed* 20:75–89, 1992.

2. Gibbons LW, Cooper KH, Meyer BM, et al: The acute cardiac risk of strenuous exercise. *JAMA* 244:1799–1801, 1980.
3. Noakes TD, Opie LH, Rose AG: Marathon running and immunity to coronary heart disease: Fact versus fiction. *Clin Sports Med* 3:527–543, 1984.
4. Thompson PD, Funk EJ, Carleton RA, et al: Incidence of death during jogging in Rhode Island from 1975 through 1980. *JAMA* 247:2535–2538, 1982.
5. Siscovick DS, Weiss NS, Fletcher RH, et al: The incidence of primary cardiac arrest during vigorous exercise. *N Engl J Med* 311:874–877, 1984.
6. Waller BF: Exercise-related sudden death in young (age <30 years) and old (age >30 years) conditioned subjects. In Wenger NK (ed): *Exercise and the Heart*, ed 2. FA Davis, Philadelphia 1985, pp 9–73.
7. Maron BJ, Roberts WC, McAllister HA Jr, et al: Sudden death in young athletes. *Circulation* 62:218–229, 1980.
8. Maron BJ, Shirani J, Mueller FO, et al: Cardiovascular causes of "athletic field" deaths: Analysis of sudden death in 84 competitive athletes (abstract). *Circulation* 88:I–50, 1993.
9. Corrado D, Thiene G, Cocco P, et al: Non-atherosclerotic coronary artery disease and sudden death in the young. *Br Heart J* 68:601–607, 1992.
10. Burke AP, Farb A, Virmani R, et al: Sports-related and non-sports-related sudden cardiac death in young adults. *Am Heart J* 121:568–575, 1991.
11. Burke AP, Subramanian R, Smialek J, et al: Nonatherosclerotic narrowing of the atrioventricular node artery and sudden death. *J Am Coll Cardiol* 21:117–122, 1993.
12. Morales AR, Romanelli R, Boucek RJ: The mural left anterior descending coronary artery, strenuous exercise and sudden death. *Circulation* 62:230–237, 1980.
13. McKenna WJ, Thiene G, Nava A, et al on behalf of the Task Force of the Working Group on Myocardial and Pericardial Disease of the European Society of Cardiology and the Scientific Council on Cardiomyopathies of the International Society and Federation of Cardiology, supported by the Schoepfer Association: Diagnosis of arrhythmogenic right ventricular dysplasia/cardiomyopathy. *Br Heart J* 71:215–218, 1994.
14. Furlanello F, Bettini R, Bertoldi A, et al: Arrhythmia patterns in athletes with arrhythmogenic right ventricular dysplasia. *Eur Heart J* 10(Suppl D):16–19, 1989.
15. Thiene G, Nava A, Corrado D, et al: Right ventricular cardiomyopathy and sudden death in young people. *N Engl J Med* 318:129–133, 1988.
16. Corrado D, Thiene G, Nava A, et al: Sudden death in young competitive athletes: Clinicopathologic correlations in 22 cases. *Am J Med* 89:588–596, 1990.
17. Zehender M, Meinertz T, Keul J, et al: ECG variants and cardiac arrhythmias in athletes: Clinical relevance and prognostic importance. *Am Heart J* 119:1378–1391, 1990.
18. Mont L, Seixas T, Brugada P, et al: Clinical and electrophysiologic characteristics of exercise-related idiopathic ventricular tachycardia. *Am J Cardiol* 68:897–900, 1991.
19. Furlanello F, Bertoldi A, Bettini R, et al: Life-threatening tachyarrhythmias in athletes. *PACE* 15:1403–1411, 1992.
20. Wiedermann CJ, Becker AE, Hopferwieser T, et al: Sudden death in a young competitive athlete with Wolff-Parkinson-White syndrome. *Eur Heart J* 8:651–655, 1987.
21. Velebit V, Podrid P, Lown B, et al: Aggravation and provocation of ventricular arrhythmias by antiarrhythymic drugs. *Circulation* 65:886–894, 1982.
22. Kloner RA, Hale S, Alker K, et al: The effects of acute and chronic cocaine use on the heart. *Circulation* 85:407–419, 1992.
23. Virmani R, Robinowitz M, McAllister HA Jr: Nontraumatic death in joggers. A series of 30 patients at autopsy. *Am J Med* 72:874–881, 1982.
24. Maron BJ, Gardin JM, Flack JM, et al: How common is hypertrophic cardiomyopathy?:

Echocardiographically identified prevalence in a general population of young adults (the CARDIA Study) (abstract). *Circulation* 88:I–452, 1993.
25. Pelliccia A, Spataro A, Maron BJ: Prospective echocardiographic screening for coronary artery anomalies in 1360 elite competitive athletes. *Am J Cardiol* 72:978–979, 1993.
26. Click RL, Holmes DR, Vlietstra RE, et al and the participants of the Coronary Artery Surgery Study (CASS): Anomalous coronary arteries: Location, degree of atherosclerosis and effect on survival—a report from the Coronary Artery Surgery Study. *J Am Coll Cardiol* 13:531–537, 1989.
27. Diamond GA, Forrester JS: Analysis of probability as an aid in the clinical diagnosis of coronary artery disease. *N Engl J Med* 300:1350–1358, 1979.
28. Epstein SE, Maron BJ: Sudden death and the competitive athlete: Perspectives on preparticipation screening studies. *J Am Coll Cardiol* 7:220–230, 1986.
29. Sakaguchi S, Shultz JJ, Remole SC, et al: Syncope associated with exercise, a manifestation of neurally mediated syncope. *Am J Cardiol* 75:476–481, 1995.
30. Maron BJ, Lipson LC, Roberts WC, et al: "Malignant" hypertrophic cardiomyopathy: Identification of a subgroup of families with unusually frequent premature death. *Am J Cardiol* 41:1133–1140, 1978.
31. Maron BJ, Nichols PF III, Pickle LW, et al: Patterns of inheritance in hypertrophic cardiomyopathy: Assessment by M-mode and two-dimensional echocardiography. *Am J Cardiol* 53:1087–1094, 1984.
32. Laurent M, Descaves C, Biron Y, et al: Familial form of arrhythmogenic right ventricular dysplasia. *Am Heart J* 113:827–829, 1987.
33. Nava A, Thiene G, Canciani B, et al: Familial occurrence of right ventricular dysplasia. A study involving nine families. *J Am Coll Cardiol* 12:1222–1228, 1988.
34. Romano C, Gemme G, Pongiglione R: Aritmie cardia che rare dell'eta pediatricia. *Clin Pediatr* (Phila) 45:656–683, 1963.
35. Ward OC: New familial cardiac syndrome in children. *J Irish Med Assoc* 54:103–106, 1964.
36. Stamler J, Wentworth D, Neaton JD: Is the risk between serum cholesterol and risk of premature death from coronary heart disease continuous and graded? *JAMA* 256:2823–2828, 1986.
37. Chaitman BR, Bourassa MG, Davis K, et al: Angiographic prevalence of high-risk coronary artery disease in patient subgroups (CASS). *Circulation* 64:360–367, 1981.
38. Pryor DB, Harrell FE, Lee KL, et al: Estimating the likelihood of significant coronary artery disease. *Am J Med* 75:771–780, 1983.
39. Huston TP, Puffer JC, Rodney WM: The athletic heart syndrome. *N Engl J Med* 313:24–32, 1985.
40. Maron BJ, Leon MB, Swain JA, et al: Prospective identification by two-dimensional echocardiography of anomalous origin of the left main coronary from the right sinus of Valsalva. *Am J Cardiol* 68:140–142, 1991.
41. Maron BJ: Structural features of the athlete heart as defined by echocardiography. *J Am Coll Cardiol* 7:190–203, 1986.
42. Pelliccia A, Maron BJ, Spataro A, et al: The upper limit of physiologic cardiac hypertrophy in highly trained elite athletes. *N Engl J Med* 324:295–301, 1991.
43. Spirito P, Pelliccia A, Proschan MA, et al: Morphology of the "Athletes heart" assessed by echocardiography in 947 elite athletes representing 27 sports. *Am J Cardiol* 74:802–806, 1994.
44. Lewis JF, Spirito P, Maron BJ: Usefulness of Doppler echocardiographic assessment of diastolic filling in distinguishing "athletes heart" from hypertrophic cardiomyopathy. *Br Heart J* 68:296–300, 1992.

45. Douglas PS, Berman GO, O'Toole ML, et al: Prevalence of multivalvular regurgitation in athletes. *Am J Cardiol* 64:209–212, 1989.
46. Maron BJ, Spirito P, Wesley Y, et al: Development and progression of left ventricular hypertrophy in children with hypertrophic cardiomyopathy. *N Engl J Med* 315:610–614, 1986.
47. Maron BJ, Bodison SA, Wesley YE, et al: Results of screening a large group of intercollegiate competitive athletes for cardiovascular disease. *J Am Coll Cardiol* 10:1214–1221, 1987.
48. Lewis JF, Maron BJ, Diggs JA, et al: Preparticipation echocardiographic screening for cardiovascular disease in a large, predominantly black population of collegiate athletes. *Am J Cardiol* 64:1029–1033, 1989.
49. Takaro T, Hultgren HN, Lipton MJ, et al: The VA cooperative randomized study of surgery for coronary arterial occlusive disease. II. Subgroup with significant left main lesions. *Circulation* 54(Suppl III):III107–III117, 1976.
50. European Coronary Surgery Study Group: Long-term results of prospective randomized study of coronary artery bypass surgery in stable angina pectoris. *Lancet* 2:1173–1180, 1982.
51. Passamani E, Davis KB, Gillespie MJ, et al: A randomized trial of coronary artery bypass surgery: Survival of patients with a low ejection fraction. *N Engl J Med* 312:1665–1671, 1985.
52. CASS Principal Investigators and Their Associates. Myocardial infarction and mortality in the Coronary Artery Surgery Study (CASS) randomized trial. *N Engl J Med* 310:750–758, 1984.
53. Varnauskas E, European Coronary Surgery Study Group: Survival, myocardial infarction, and employment status in a prospective randomized study of coronary bypass surgery. *Circulation* 72(Suppl 5):V90–V101, 1985.
54. Mock MB, Fisher LD, Holmes DR Jr, et al: Comparison of effects of medical and surgical therapy on survival in severe angina pectoris and two-vessel coronary artery disease with and without left ventricular dysfunction: A Coronary Artery Surgery Study Registry Study. *Am J Cardiol* 61:1198–1203, 1988.
55. Pepine CP, Cohn PF, Deedwania PC, et al for the Assist Study Group: Effects of treatment on outcome in mildly symptomatic patients with ischemia during daily life. The Atenolol Silent Ischemia Study (ASIST). *Circulation* 90:762–768, 1994.
56. Steering Committee of the Physicians' Health Study Research Group: Final report on the aspirin component of the ongoing Physicians' Health Study. *N Engl J Med* 321:129–135, 1989.
57. Gianrossi R, Detrano R, Mulvihill D, et al: Exercise-induced ST depression in the diagnosis of coronary artery disease: A meta-analysis. *Circulation* 80:87–98, 1989.
58. Epstein SE, Quyyumi AA, Bonow RO: Myocardial ischemia—silent or symptomatic. *N Engl J Med* 318:1038–1043, 1988.
59. Bruce RA, Fisher LD, Hossack KF: Validation of exercise-enhanced risk assessment of coronary heart disease events: Longitudinal changes in incidence in Seattle community practice. *J Am Coll Cardiol* 5:875–881, 1985.
60. Multiple Risk Factor Intervention Trial Research Group: Exercise electrocardiogram and coronary heart disease mortality in the Multiple Risk Factor Intervention Trial. *Am J Cardiol* 55:16–24, 1985.
61. Ekelund LG, Suchindran CM, McMahon RP, et al: Coronary heart disease morbidity and mortality in hypercholesterolemic men predicted from an exercise test: The Lipid Research Clinics Coronary Primary Prevention Trial. *J Am Coll Cardiol* 14:556–563, 1989.

62. Schlant RC, Blomqvist CG, Brandenburg RO, et al: Guidelines for exercise testing. A report of the American College of Cardiology/American Heart Association Task Force on assessment of cardiovascular procedures (subcommittee on exercise testing). *J Am Coll Cardiol* 8:725–738, 1986.
63. Breen JF, Sheedy PF, Schwartz RF, et al: Coronary artery calcification detected with ultrafast CT as an indication of coronary artery disease. *Radiology* 185:435–439, 1992.
64. Powell KE, Thompson PD, Casperson CJ, et al: Physical activity and the incidence of coronary heart disease. *Ann Rev Public Health* 8:253–287, 1987.
65. Siscovick DS, Weiss NS, Fletcher RJ, et al: The incidence of primary cardiac arrest during vigorous exercise. *N Engl J Med* 311:874–877, 1984.
66. Fletcher GF, Balady G, Froelicher VF, et al: Exercise standards. A statement for healthcare professionals from the American Heart Association. *Circulation* 91:580–615, 1995.
67. Siscovick DS, Ekelund LG, Johnson JL, et al: Sensitivity of exercise electrocardiography for acute cardiac events during moderate and strenuous physical activity. The Lipids Research Clinics Coronary Primary Prevention Trial. *Arch Intern Med* 151:325–330, 1991.
68. American College of Sports Medicine: *Guidelines for Exercise Testing and Prescription,* ed 4. Philadelphia, Lea and Febiger, 1991.
69. Pate RR, Pratt M, Blair SN, et al: Physical activity and public health. A recommendation from the Centers for Disease Control and Prevention and the American College of Sports Medicine. *JAMA* 273:402–407, 1995.
70. Maron BJ, Mitchell JH: Bethesda Conference Report. 26th Bethesda Conference: Recommendations for determining eligibility for competition in athletes with cardiovascular abnormalities. *J Am Coll Cardiol* 24:845–899, 1994.
71. Maron BJ, Klues HG: Surviving competitive athletics with hypertrophic cardiomyopathy. *Am J Cardiol* 73:1098–1104, 1994.
72. Hossack KF, Hartwig R: Cardiac arrest associated with supervised cardiac rehabilitation. *J Cardiac Rehb* 2:402–408, 1982.
73. Sullivan MJ, Higginbotham MB, Cobb FR: Exercise training in patients with severe left ventricular dysfunction. Hemodynamic and metabolic effects. *Circulation* 78:506–515, 1988.
74. McKelvie RS, Teo KK, McCartney N, et al: Effects of exercise training in patients with congestive heart failure: A critical review. *J Am Coll Cardiol* 25:789–796, 1995.
75. Squires RW, Muri AJ, Anderson LJ, et al: Weight training during Phase II (early outpatient) cardiac rehabilitation: Heart rate and blood pressure responses. *J Cardiopulm Rehab* 11:360–364, 1991.

♦ CHAPTER SIX ♦

EXERCISE GUIDELINES FOR PATIENTS WITH CONGENITAL CARDIOVASCULAR DISORDERS

Marla A. Mendelson, M.D.

INTRODUCTION

Adults born with congenital heart disease constitute a unique patient population. As adults, they present therapeutic challenges that may be unique to the individual patient. The adult is often a survivor of multiple complex surgeries that restore physiology but not necessarily normal anatomic structure. Also, patients may present initially as adults diagnosed with congenital heart disease because of the advances in diagnostic techniques. The physician making recommendations regarding participation in sports and exercise must consider the original cardiac lesion, type of repair, and sequelae of surgery. Exercise, ranging from recreational sports and aerobic conditioning to competitive sport participation, will vary. Therefore, the exercise prescription must be individualized based on both the type of exercise and the patient's hemodynamic status.

Exercise can have multiple meanings and definitions. When a patient with congenital cardiovascular disorders presents for exercise recommendations, it is particularly important to specify the type of exercise or sport involved. *Competitive athletics* are characterized by sustained activity with superimposed emotional pressure and a training commitment, and therefore carry different considerations than recreational athletics. *Recreational athletics* may also involve competition and require training but may not have the same emotional pressures.[1] Certain sports may have a risk of collision which is important to consider, for example, if a patient is anticoagulated.

The physiologic type of exercise is also important to consider for the person with congenital heart disease. Dynamic (isotonic) exercise occurs when muscular force is exerted in association with changes in muscle length. The result is an increase in oxygen consumption, stroke volume, cardiac output, and systolic blood pressure. Diastolic blood pressure usually remains unchanged as peripheral resistance falls. By contrast, static (isometric) exercise occurs when muscular force is exerted without a change in muscle length.[1] During static exercise, there is a sudden increase in systolic, diastolic, and mean arterial blood pressures and a smaller increase in oxygen consumption and cardiac output. This type of exercise may be associated with a Valsalva maneuver, which for some patients may be deleterious.

The duration, frequency, and setting in which exercise will occur should also be identified by the patient before recommendations are made. Specific types of exercise are classified as low, moderate or high in intensity based on the activity required and are further divided into static or dynamic activities (see Appendix 1 for a complete classification of physical activities).

The adult with congenital heart disease who has undergone surgical correction will most likely have had a form of palliation or repair to reestablish physiologic, if not anatomic, integrity. For example, the patient with a patent ductus arteriosus may truly be cured of congenital heart disease, but patients born with all other lesions may have residua or sequelae that may impact on their functional status. Examples of surgical residua may include prosthetic material used in conduits, patches or valves; residual shunting; or residual elevations in pulmonary arterial pressures. The sequelae of surgery may be myocardial dysfunction and/or arrhythmias due to the type of surgical repair. These sequelae and residua may constitute contraindications to exercise, as detailed in Table 6-1.

Before recommendations for exercise are made, the patient should undergo a complete evaluation by a physician familiar with congenital heart disease as manifest in the adult. Chapters 4 and 5 discuss the medical evaluation of patients with cardiovascular disease who are about to begin an exercise program. Patients with congenital heart disease may require more advanced testing (electrophysiologic testing, left- and/or right-heart catheterization, transesophageal echocardiography, etc.), depending on the disorder and its severity.

CONGENITAL VALVULAR HEART DISEASE

CASE EXAMPLE

Patient History and Examination

A 25-year-old male presents with a history of bicuspid aortic valve. He is 50 lb overweight and wishes to begin a weight loss and exercise program. He is

TABLE 6-1. Contraindications to exercise in the adult with congenital heart disease

Cardiac Lesion	Clinical Contraindication
Aortic stenosis	Severe stenosis (≥50 mm Hg*) Exertional syncope Severe left ventricular hypertrophy
Aortic insufficiency	Severe symptomatic aortic insufficiency
Atrial septal defect, unrepaired	Marked cyanosis Eisenmenger's syndrome Large right-to-left shunt
Ventricular septal defect, unrepaired	Pulmonary hypertension Ventricular dysfunction
Patent ductus arteriosus, unrepaired	Large shunt with pulmonary hypertension
Patent ductus arteriosus, repaired	Residual pulmonary hypertension
Ebstein's anomaly	Severe form of anomaly Cyanosis
Marfan syndrome	Severe aortic insufficiency Aortic root dilatation
Congenital prolonged Q-T syndrome	Symptomatic ventricular arrhythmias Family history of sudden death Prolonged Q-T interval
Anomalous origin of the left coronary artery	Angina Myocardial infarction Sudden death

*Instantaneous systolic pressure gradient.

currently asymptomatic. On examination, his blood pressure is 120/70 mm Hg, with a heart rate of 76 beats per minute. His lungs are clear, and he has normal first and second heart sounds with a regular rhythm. He has an ejection click and a harsh 3/6 systolic murmur radiating to his carotids.

The electrocardiogram is normal, and echocardiography reveals left ventricular wall thickness at the upper limit of normal. On a Bruce protocol stress test, the patient completes 9 min of exercise without symptoms. He has moderately severe aortic stenosis with a peak instantaneous pressure gradient of 30 mm Hg by Doppler echocardiography. There is no evidence of marked left ventricular hypertrophy.

Exercise Recommendation

Since there is no evidence of left ventricular hypertrophy, the patient may consider activities with low static demands and low to moderate dynamic demands (groups IA or IB, Appendix 1), such as doubles tennis, softball, or volleyball.

Aortic Valve Disease

BISCUSPID AORTIC VALVE

One of the most common congenital heart lesions in the adult is a bicuspid aortic valve. This can be a malformed trileaflet valve, which may result in isolated aortic stenosis, isolated aortic insufficiency, or a combination of both. It is often undetected until adulthood and carries a potential risk of endocarditis. It may be associated with other congenital lesions, most notably coarctation of the aorta. The patient may have had a coarctation repaired as a child, but may have residual aortic stenosis or insufficiency due to a bicuspid aortic valve.

AORTIC STENOSIS

The exercise capacity in patients with aortic stenosis is based solely on the degree of stenosis and left ventricular function. These recommendations also apply to patients with subaortic and supravalvular aortic stenosis. Symptoms may include fatigue, lightheadedness, syncope, or chest pain on exercise.[2,3] If symptoms are present, the patient should undergo stress testing and possibly cardiac catheterization. The patient at risk for sudden death during exercise has left ventricular hypertrophy, exertional syncope, chest pain, or dyspnea.[2]

The patient with mild aortic stenosis (≤20 mm Hg peak instantaneous systolic pressure gradient) may participate in all sports if asymptomatic, has a normal echocardiogram, and a normal stress test.[2] Patients with moderate aortic stenosis (21–49 mm Hg gradient) should be restricted to low to moderate static exercise with low dynamic demands (groups IA, IB, or IIA) if asymptomatic, with minimal left ventricular hypertrophy and a normal stress test.[2] Higher-intensity static exercise should be discouraged because it will increase ventricular afterload.[1] Patients with severe aortic stenosis (≥80 mm Hg gradient) should not participate in competitive sports.[1,2] These patients are at risk for sudden death, from either arrhythmia or outflow tract obstruction, and may require valve replacement, valvotomy, or valvuloplasty prior to participation in exercise.[2]

After intervention, the same criteria apply based on the level of residual stenosis. The major risk in patients who have received a prosthetic valve for aortic stenosis or insufficiency is that they require therapeutic anticoagulation. They should avoid sports that would increase their risk of head injuries, such as downhill skiing, bunge jumping, boxing, motorcycle racing, or any sport with a potential for bodily collision.

AORTIC INSUFFICIENCY

The patient with aortic insufficiency is at risk for progressive ventricular dilatation and may experience angina, syncope, arrhythmias, or sudden death with exercise.[2,4] Echocardiography helps assess the extent of valvular regurgitation, as well as left ventricular and aortic root size. The patient with mild aortic insufficiency and a normal left ventricle without peripheral signs of aortic insufficiency may participate in sports.[5] The individual with moderate aortic insufficiency with peripheral signs, left ventricular enlargement, and preserved systolic function may also participate in sports.[5] In the setting of severe aortic insufficiency with left ventricular enlargement and dysfunction, participation in sports is not recommended.[5]

Pulmonic Valve Disease

PULMONIC STENOSIS

The patient with mild pulmonic stenosis (<25 mm Hg gradient) and a normal electrocardiogram may have unrestricted athletic activity.[1,2] patients with moderate obstruction (25–50 mm Hg gradient) may tolerate competitive sports but should be limited if there is electrocardiographic evidence of right ventricular hypertrophy.[2] The patient with severe pulmonic stenosis (>50 mm Hg gradient) should be limited to low-intensity exercise (group IA) if there is evidence of impaired right ventricular function.[1,2] This patient should be considered for balloon dilatation of the valve. After balloon dilatation, the residual gradient and pulmonic valve insufficiency should determine athletic recommendations.[1] There may be a return to activity 1 month after balloon valvotomy or 3 months after surgery.[2]

PULMONARY VALVE REGURGITATION

Pulmonic regurgitation after balloon valvotomy or tetralogy of Fallot repair may be congenital or residual. Patients should not be restricted if their exercise tolerance is normal.[1] They should be assessed periodically for the degree of regurgitation. If regurgitation increases or there is evidence of ventricular compromise, further evaluation may be required.[1]

SEPTAL DEFECTS

CASE EXAMPLE

Patient History and Examination

A 24-year-old female presents with a history of a heart murmur. She seeks advice regarding playing tennis with her friends. She states that she has had chest discomfort and lightheadedness when walking rapidly and notes palpitations. On examination her blood pressure is 100/60 mmHg and her pulse is irregularly irregular at a rate of 100 beats per minute. Her lungs are clear. She has a right ventricular heave. The rhythm is irregularly irregular. She has a wide, fixed splitting of the second heart sound with a loud pulmonic component. There is a midsystolic ejection murmur at the second left interspace. There is a holosystolic murmur that increases with inspiration and an early diastolic murmur. There is mild clubbing and cyanosis of her fingers and toes. These findings are consistent with an atrial septal defect with pulmonary hypertension. There is evidence of shunt reversal (right to left).

Exercise Recommendation

The ability of patients with septal defects to exercise is often determined by the level of pulmonary vascular resistance. When pulmonary arterial pressures are elevated, cyanosis may increase with exercise and there is an increased risk of sudden death. This patient should avoid exercise and undergo further evaluation.

Atrial Septal Defect

The adult with an atrial septal defect that has gone previously undetected is most likely to have a secundum atrial septal defect. These defects at the site of the fossa ovalis may vary in size and have associated right ventricular volume overload. If they are uncomplicated, the adult patient may have already participated in exercise.[1] If they are small and the pulmonary artery pressures are normal, the patient should not be restricted.[2] Closure of the atrial septal defect may be recommended, as there is a risk of paradoxical emboli. The patient with mild pulmonary hypertension or right-to-left shunting should be restricted to low-intensity activities (group IA).[2] Exercise is prohibited in the setting of marked cyanosis, Eisenmenger's complex, or a large right-to-left shunt.[2] Theoretically, underwater diving may pose a risk in the patient with an unrepaired atrial septal defect.

Postoperative patients without residual right ventricular enlargement, shunt, or pulmonary hypertension who have a complete repair may participate in exercise without restriction after 6 months if they remain asymptomatic, without arrhythmias or ventricular dysfunction.[2] However, if there is residual pulmonary arterial hypertension (>20 mm Hg) and evidence of conduction abnormalities or atrial arrhythmias, exercise should be limited to low-intensity types (group IA).[1,2,6]

Ventricular Septal Defect

Ventricular septal defects most commonly present in adults as a defect either on the membranous septum or on the muscular septum. The membranous defect may involve the aortic valve, which may prolapse into the defect, resulting in aortic insufficiency. Ventricular septal defects are usually detected by physical examination and confirmed by Doppler echocardiography. A small defect associated with normal pulmonary vascular resistance allows unlimited activity and participation in competitive sports.[1,2] The degree of pulmonary vascular resistance will dictate whether the patient can participate in sports. If resistance is elevated, the patient may be restricted to low-intensity activities (group IA).[2]

After closure of a ventricular septal defect in childhood, there may be residual shunting, cardiomegaly, myocardial dysfunction, or elevated pulmonary vascular resistance.[1] If any of these conditions are present, further investigation by stress testing and possibly cardiac catheterization is warranted.[2] After closure, if there is no evidence of arrhythmias and a small residual shunt with normal ventricular size and function, the patient's activity can be unrestricted after 6 months.[1,2] The patient with a moderate or large shunt after surgery as a child can participate in low-intensity activity (group IA), but definitive repair should be considered.[2] Sports are prohibited if there is significant pulmonary hypertension or ventricular dysfunction.[2]

Patent Ductus Arteriosus

The asymptomatic adult with a small, unrepaired patent ductus arteriosus, normal heart size, and normal pulmonary vascular resistance may participate in sports.[1,2] If there is a large shunt with cardiomegaly and pulmonary pressures are elevated, the patient may require intervention and should not participate in sports.[2] After repair, if the patient is asymptomatic, has a normal examination, and is without pulmonary hypertension, participation in sports is permitted.[2] The patient with residual preliminary hypertension should be restricted.[1,2]

CYANOTIC CONGENITAL HEART DISEASE

CASE EXAMPLE

Patient History and Examination

A 30-year-old male who was born with tetralogy of Fallot underwent a primary repair at age 5 years. He has been able to exercise modestly without problems but now wishes to train for the next decathlon. He is asymptomatic at rest or with jogging. On examination, his blood pressure is 120/70 mm Hg, and his heart rate is 68 beats per minute and regular. His lungs are clear. He has a very soft diastolic murmur at the left upper sternal border.

The patient undergoes two-dimensional and Doppler echocargiography, which reveal an intact septal patch without a residual shunt and normal right ventricular morphology with minimal pulmonic regurgitation. His 24-hr ambulatory electrocardiogram and Bruce protocol stress test are both normal and without evidence of arrhythmia.

Exercise Recommendations

The patient can be cleared to train for the decathlon, but he should return for periodic evaluation.

Adults with cyanotic congenital heart disease who have not undergone definitive repair will have self-limited activity and will participate only in low-intensity exercise. Their oxygen saturation may decline further with exercise. The patient with residual cyanosis after repair or palliation can participate in low-intensity activities if the oxygen saturation is greater than 80%, there are no symptomatic arrhythmias, and ventricular function is adequate.[2] Therefore, these recommendations will focus on the adult who has undergone palliation or repair.

Tetralogy of Fallot

The adult with tetralogy of Fallot born with an overriding aorta, a large ventricular septal defect, pulmonary outflow tract narrowing, and right ventricular hypertrophy usually has undergone palliation or repair. The adult with uncorrected tetralogy of Fallot will be cyanotic because of mixing of blood, may be limited in daily activities, and should avoid static exercise. The patient who has optimal anatomy for correction and had corrective surgery early in childhood may be able to participate in sports without risks, although exercise capacity and stress response may be abnormal.[7]

Postoperative patients are at risk for residual left-to-right shunting, pulmonic insufficiency, right ventricular dysfunction, syncope, ventricular arrhythmia, and sudden death.[1,2,8] These patients should be assessed with exercise testing and echocardiography, as well as ambulatory electrocardiography.

After repair, the patient may participate in all sports if right-sided pressures are normal, right ventricular volume overload is mild, and no residual shunting occurs.[1,2] There should be no resting or exercise-induced arrhythmias.[1,2] The patient with palliative shunting for tetralogy of Fallot who has not had a definitive repair will probably have decreased oxygen saturation, which should be monitored during exercise to see if a further decline occurs.[1] If a decrease does occur, participation in exercise should be limited. Low-intensity activity (group IA) is recommended for the patient with severe residual pulmonic insufficiency, right ventricular hypertension, or arrhythmias.[2]

Transposition of the Great Arteries

The adult with transposition of the great arteries has the aorta arising from the right ventricle and the pulmonary artery receiving blood from the left ventricle. At the time of this writing most adults with this condition will have had an atrial switch operation earlier in life (Mustard or Senning). There is a younger population of patients who will have had the arterial switch operation, but these comments are limited to those adults who have undergone the Mustard or Senning procedure. These surgeries involve redirecting the incoming blood flow to the appropriate ventricle. This requires extensive atrial surgery, and therefore the survivors are at risk for development of atrial arrhythmias and junctional rhythms. There may be residual abnormalities in systemic (right) ventricular function, pulmonic stenosis, pulmonary hypertension, tricuspid insufficiency, ventricular arrhythmias, or left ventricular abnormalities.[9]

To participate in low to moderate static activity or low dynamic activity, there should be a normal cardiac silhouette on chest radiography, no atrial or ventricular arrhythmias, no history of syncope, and a normal stress test.[2] The stress test is also useful to ensure that arrhythmias are not provoked by exercise.[10]

The patient born with congenitally corrected transposition of the great arteries (ventricular inversion) is at risk for atrioventricular valve abnormalities, ventricular septal defect, and atrioventricular heart block.[2] There may be full participation in sports if heart size and function are normal, there is a nearly normal stress test, no symptoms, and no evidence of arrhythmias on monitoring.[2] These patients should have periodic assessment of systemic (right) ventricular function, which may remain subnormal.[1]

The Postoperative Fontan Operation

The Fontan operation is used for the patient born with a single ventricle or tricuspid atresia to direct vena caval flow to the pulmonary arteries. The ventricle becomes solely a systemic ventricle effectively separating the venous and arterial circulations. Although exercise tolerance may improve after surgery, it may remain subnormal and there may be an age-related decline in exercise performance.[11,12] Residual sequelae may include valve regurgitation and abnormal ventricular function.[1,2] Low-intensity activities (group IA) may be permitted if ventricular function and oxygen saturation are normal at rest and during exercise.[2]

Ebstein's Anomaly

Ebstein's anomaly varies in severity, based on the extent of atrialization of the right ventricle with downward displacement of the tricuspid valve, interatrial shunting, cyanosis, and tricuspid regurgitation. The adult with unrepaired Ebstein's anomaly most likely has a milder form of disease but should undergo exercise stress testing prior to embarking on an exercise program.[2] There is a risk of arrhythmias related to an underlying Wolff-Parkinson-White syndrome. Participation in sports is permitted if the patient is acyanotic, has a normal heart size, and has no evidence of arrhythmias.[2] Low-intensity activity (group IA) is permitted if tricuspid regurgitation is moderate but arrhythmias are absent. Exercise is prohibited with severe Ebstein's anomaly.[2]

After childhood repair, there should be assessment with ambulatory electrocardiographic monitoring and stress testing. Low-intensity activity (group IA) is recommended if tricuspid regurgitation is mild, heart size is normal, and there is no evidence of arrhythmias.[2]

AORTIC DISEASE

CASE EXAMPLE

Patient History and Examination

A 12-year-old boy is brought to you by his mother for a preparticipation physical examination before trying out for his school's basketball team. Because of his tall stature, his mother worries about the possibility of his having Marfan syndrome. There is no family history of Marfan syndrome, nor is there a family history of sudden or premature cardiac death. The patient is symptom free.

On examination the patient is found to be 70 in. tall, weighs 135 lb, and has an arm span of 73 in. an upper body length of 30 in., and a lower body length of 40 in. He has a positive thumb sign and positive wrist sign. No other musculoskeletal abnormalities are noted. He has had a recent eye examination by an ophthalmologist, which was normal. His physical examination is unremarkable, with the exception of a soft grade II systolic murmur which is heard best over the left upper sternal border, diminishes on standing, does not change with squatting or Valsalva manuever, and does not radiate to the carotids. Echocardiography reveals no valvular abnormalities and no evidence of aortic root dilatation.

Exercise Recommendations

The patient fails to meet the diagnostic criteria for Marfan syndrome, although he does have musculoskeletal abnormalities suggestive of the disorder. The patient has a nonpathologic "innocent" murmur (see Chapter 4). He can be cleared for participation in basketball, but should be followed closely for the development of other findings consistent with Marfan syndrome in the event that they develop as the patient ages.

Marfan Syndrome

Marfan syndrome is an inherited abnormality of the aorta that carries the risk of progressive aortic dilatation often resulting in aortic dissection or rupture. These patients may myxomatous mitral valve prolapse with mitral regurgitation. Patients with aortic dilatation should have periodic echocardiograms and often computed tomography studies to evaluate the aortic root. If the aortic root is less than 4 cm and is not dilated, and if there is no family history of sudden death or severe mitral regurgitation, patients may participate in low to moderate static activities with low dynamic demands (groups IA and IIA; see Appendix 1), such as bowling, golf, and archery.[2] If aortic root dilatation is present, then only low-intensity activities (group IA) should be recommended.[2] Activities with collision risk should be avoided. Periodic echocardiography is recommended to detect aortic root dilatation.[2]

Coarctation of the Aorta

Coarctation of the aorta in the adult usually involves narrowing of the aorta distal to the origin of the left subclavian artery. These patients have extensive collateral flow through bronchial arteries resulting in the characteristic rib notching seen on chest radiography. The major cardiac risks include endarteritis, hypertension, and aortic dissection. There is a strong association with a bicuspid aortic valve (see the preceding recommendations for exercise in the presence of bicuspid aortic valve). The severity of coarctation can be established by transthoracic or transesophageal Doppler echocardiography and can be detected by magnetic resonance imaging. If coarctation is present without large collaterals or aortic root dilatation, the exercise stress is normal, and the gradient between the arm and leg blood pressures is <20 mm Hg, the patient may participate in all sports.[2] Stress testing is particularly important in postoperative patients because these patients have abnormal vascular activity and may have a pronounced systolic blood pressure elevation during exercise. If the systolic blood pressure during exercise is less than 230 mm Hg, and there is <20 mm Hg gradient between the arm and leg pressures at rest, the patient may participate in activities.[2] If the arm/leg pressure gradient is >20 mm Hg or there is exercise-induced hypertension, low-intensity activity (group IA) is recommended.[2]

Patients who underwent repair as a child may have a mild residual gradient, left ventricular hypertrophy, and systemic hypertension; there may also be pronounced systolic blood pressure increases during exercise.[13,14] These patients should be initially evaluated for left ventricular function using chest radiography and stress testing.[2] Magnetic resonance imaging is useful in a patient who has undergone balloon angioplasty to detect the presence of an aneurysm. Six months after repair, if the arm/leg pressure gradient is ≤20 mm Hg and there is a normal peak systolic blood pressure with exercise, the patient may participate in activity but should be restricted from activity with collision risk for approximately 1 year. If aneurysmal dilatation of the aorta is present, the patient should be restricted to low-intensity activity (group IA) and avoid static activity.[2]

ARRHYTHMIAS

The arrhythmias discussed here will be only those that complicate congenital heart disease or may be residua or sequelae of congenital heart disease surgery.[15,16] The same evaluation, including a 12-lead electrocardiogram, echocardiography, stress testing, and 24-hr ambulatory electrocardiographic monitoring, preferably during activity, is recommended. These patients should also be reevaluated after training.[12] In general, for arrhythmias during which the ventricular rates are comparable to the tachycardic response of the exercise, the patient may continue to exercise.[15] Specific arrhythmias will be discussed.

Atrial Flutter

The risk of atrial flutter is progression to 1:1 conduction. Stress testing will determine the response to exercise and guide therapy and further exercise recommendations. The patient on medications to treat atrial flutter with a normal heart may participate in low-intensity activity (group IA) and may be considered for full participation in all sports if he or she has no atrial flutter for 3–6 months.[15] The patient with underlying structural heart disease may participate in low-intensity activity if asymptomatic for more than 6 months.[15]

Atrial Fibrillation

After evaluation, the patient with atrial fibrillation and structural heart disease with an adequate ventricular rate should have limited exercise, depending on the nature of the underlying heart disease.[2] If the ventricular rate with exercise is similar to the expected sinus tachycardic response, exercise is permitted.[15] These patients are often anticoagulated and should avoid sports or activities that have the risk of bodily collision or severe injury.[2]

Supraventricular Tachycardia

The patient who has exercise-induced supraventricular tachycardia but who is asymptomatic may participate in all sports.[15] If episodes occur at rest, participation in sports may be permitted after treatment has been initiated and the patient has remained asymptomatic for 6 months.[15] After ablation for a supraventricular tachycardia, the patient who remains asymptomatic for 3 to 6 months after the procedure may be cleared to participate in all sports, depending on the nature of the underlying heart disease.[15]

Wolff-Parkinson-White Syndrome

The patient without structural heart disease who remains asymptomatic may participate in all sports.[15] After ablation, the patient with a structurally normal heart who has been asymptomatic for 3 to 6 months may be cleared for participation.[15]

Ventricular Tachycardia

After thorough investigation for underlying structural heart disease, the patient may be prohibited from exercising for 6 months after the last episode if this proved to be noninducible during electrophysiologic testing. In the setting of structural heart disease, the patient may be cleared only for low-intensity activity (group IA).[15] If ventricular tachycardia is <150 beats per minute and there is no structural heart disease, there may be no increased risk.[15]

Congenital Heart Block

After complete evaluation has revealed a structurally normal heart, the heart rate is >40–50 beats per minute, and there is no evidence of ventricular tachycardia, the patient may be cleared to participate in all sports.[15,17] If ventricular ectopy, fatigue, or syncope is present, the patient should have a pacemaker placed prior to participation.[15,17] In the setting of abnormal hemodynamic status such as an intracardiac shunt, a pacemaker may need to be placed. After this is done, the patient should avoid sports with collision risk and undergo stress testing prior to participation for assessment of the heart rate response to exercise.

Congenital Prolonged Q-T Syndrome

The syndrome of congenitally prolonged Q-T interval includes a Q-T, corrected to 440 to 450 ms on a 12-lead electrocardiogram, symptoms of arrhythmia, a family history of sudden death, and other diagnostic electrocardiographic findings such as abnormal T-wave morphology.[15,18] These patients are at risk of developing ventricular tachycardia, specifically toursades des Pointes. Athletes identified with the syndrome should be prohibited from participating in sports.[15]

MISCELLANEOUS CONGENITAL DISORDERS

Coronary Artery Anomalies

There may be several anatomic variations in coronary artery origins. An anomalous right coronary artery originating from the left coronary sinus, hypoplastic arteries, or a left main artery originating from the pulmonary artery and traveling between the pulmonary trunk and aorta have been associated with sudden death during exercise.[1,2,19] These patients present with exertional angina or syncope. If the diagnosis is suspected, full evaluation should be done before the patient engages in physical activity. Cardiac catheterization will best identify the abnormal coronary anatomy, and coronary artery bypass surgery may be indicated before participation in physical activity. After surgical revascularization, the patient may be evaluated at 6 months with exercise stress testing. If there is no evidence of exercise-induced ischemia, significant ventricular dysfunction, or dangerous ventricular dysrhythmias, the patient may resume training for sports.[2]

SUMMARY

1. Recommendations regarding participation in sports must be individualized for the patient with congenital heart disease. Factors to consider include the type of activity anticipated, the original cardiac lesion, the natural history of that lesion, and the sequelae after surgical repair.
2. The 26th Bethesda Conference provides the current standards for the clearance of patient-athletes with congenital cardiovascular disease for athletic participation. With the wide array of medical and surgical treatments available to patients with congenital heart disease, many will be eligible for at least low-intensity exercise. Because of the continual advances in these treatments, new strategies and data may expand the eligibility criteria in the future.

REFERENCES

1. Kaplan S, Perloff JK: Exercise and athletics before and after surgery or interventional catheterization. In Perloff JK, Child JS (eds): *Congenital Heart Disease in Adults.* Philadelphia, WB Saunders 1991, p 166.
2. Graham TP, Bricker JT, James FW, et al: 26th Bethesda Conference. Task Force 1: Congenital Heart Disease. *J Am Coll Cardiol* 24:867–873, 1994.
3. Doyle EF, Arumugham P, Lara E, et al: Sudden death in young patients with congenital aortic stenosis. *Pediatrics* 53:481–489, 1974.
4. Dehmer GJ, Firth BG, Hillis LD, et al: Alterations in left ventricular volumes and ejection fraction at rest and during exercise in patients with aortic regurgitation. *Am J Cardiol* 48:17–27, 1981.
5. Cheitlin MD, Douglas PS, Parmley WW: 26th Bethesda Conference. Task Force 2: Acquired valvular heart disease. *J Am Coll Cardiol* 24:874–879, 1994.
6. Bink-Boelkens M Th. E, Velvis H, Homan van der Heide JJ, et al: Dysrhythmias after atrial surgery in children. *Am Heart J* 106:125–130, 1983.
7. Kaplan JD, Foster E, Redberg RF, et al: Exercise Doppler echocardiography identifies abnormal hemodynamics in adults with congenital heart disease. *Am Heart J* 127:1572–1580, 1994.
8. Garson A Jr, Gillette PC, Gutgesell HP, et al: Stress-induced ventricular arrhythmia after repair of tetralogy of Fallot. *Am J Cardiol* 46:1006–1012, 1980.
9. Graham TP Jr: Hemodynamic residua and sequelae following intraatrial repair of transposition of the great arteries: A review. *Pediatr Cardiol* 2:203–213, 1982.
10. Matthews RA, Fricker FJ, Beerman LB, et al: Exercise studies after the Mustard operation in transposition of the great arteries. *Am J Cardiol* 51:1526–1529, 1983.
11. Driscoll DJ, Danielson GK, Puga FJ, et al: Exercise tolerance and cardiorespiratory response to exercise after the Fontan operation for tricuspid atresia or functional single ventricle. *J Am Coll Cardiol* 7:1087–1094, 1986.
12. Driscoll DJ: Exercise responses in functional single ventricle before and after Fontan operation. *Prog Pediatr Cardiol* 2:44–49, 1993.
13. Pelech AN, Kartodihardjo W, Balfe JA, et al: Exercise in children before and after coarctectomy: Hemodynamic, echocardiographic, and biochemical assessment. *Am Heart J* 112:1263–1270, 1986.
14. Freed MD, Rocchini A, Rosenthal A, et al: Exercise-induced hypertension after surgical repair of coarctation of the aorta. *Am J Cardiol* 43:253–258, 1979.

15. Zipes DP, Garson A Jr: 26th Bethesda Conference. Task Force 6: Arrhythmias. *J Am Coll Cardiol* 24:892–899, 1994.
16. Vetter VL: Postoperative arrhythmias after surgery for congenital heart defects. *Cardiol Rev* 2:83–97, 1994.
17. Karpawich PP, Gillette PC, Garson A Jr, et al: Congenital complete atrioventricular block: Clinical and electrophysiologic predictors of need for pacemaker insertion. *Am J Cardiol* 48:1098–1102, 1981.
18. Garson A Jr, MacDonald D II, Fournier A, et al: The long QT syndrome in children: An international study of 287 patients. *Circulation* 887:1866–1872, 1993.
19. Maron BJ, Roberts WC, McAllister HA, et al: Sudden death in young athletes. *Circulation* 62:218–229, 1980.

♦ CHAPTER SEVEN ♦

BASIC PRINCIPLES OF EXERCISE PRESCRIPTION FOR CARDIAC PATIENTS: THE PHILOSOPHY AND ART OF EXERCISE PRESCRIPTION

Jeffrey Roitman, Ed.D.
Randal J. Thomas, M.D., M.S.

INTRODUCTION

The reasons and objectives for prescribing any therapeutic modality to patients may vary from those pertaining to return to work, facilitating return to previous functional activity levels, or allowing the completion of activities of daily living without symptoms. The objectives for prescribing exercise for cardiac patients are equally diverse. Consideration of the individual patient and appropriate personal goals and objectives should be primary when determining the appropriate dose and mode of exercise/activity for cardiac patients.

The early literature on exercise prescription and chronic adaptations to exercise training focused on eliciting a *training response*, as measured by significant increases in maximal oxygen consumption. Though this may be a pertinent goal for some individuals, perhaps even some patients, the ideal therapeutic endpoint of an exercise program may not be that simple or that direct. Consequently, new and varied approaches to exercise prescription and, thus, exercise training are being utilized.

One of these approaches relies on a *public health approach* to cardiovascular endurance exercise.[1] This approach emerged from the question "How much exercise is enough?". The answer logically depends on the answer to the question "Enough for what?" Epidemiologic researchers have attempted to find not only the frequency, duration, intensity, and total "dose" of physical activity which might lead to some protection from heart disease (i.e., related to a decrease in the death rate from coronary artery disease), but also a practical level with which many Americans could and, more important, would comply.

The recent work of Blair and others on this question seems to be particularly relevant to much of the cardiac population.[2–9] Their data shows that the inordinate reliance on the target heart rate for the purpose of inducing a training response may be misplaced for many cardiac (and other chronically diseased) patients, especially those beginning an exercise program who have little or no history of regular exercise.

That literature seems to say that, for most sedentary people (and perhaps all but the most active regular exercisers), target heart rates are of questionable value in prescribing exercise. This may be especially true for those who are inactive and have no history of regular compliance with an exercise program. Too much attention to any kind of *target heart rate* may compromise the ability of many patients to comply with the prescribed program. It appears that any activity above the accustomed level will produce some mild training effects and will also begin to produce the known health benefits of regular activity.[10,11]

The use of some type of *target heart rate range*, calculated from a treadmill test or from rating of perceived exertion (RPE) levels, can be useful and beneficial for some cardiac patients. However, the strict use of target heart rates from treadmill tests (especially if the test is inappropriate for this calculation) may not be beneficial or accurate.

For patients other than those who are symptomatic or who are ischemic by ECG standards, target heart rates are generally unimportant. In addition, most patients are not given the kind of exercise test (a maximal or symptom-limited test) that would generate heart rate information to allow calculation of a valid target heart rate range. The subsets of patients for whom target heart rates are considered important will be discussed within each patient population.

As a patient progresses in intensity and duration and complies with the appropriate frequency of exercise, increases in functional capacity will result, regardless of the application of a target heart rate. Intensity, duration, and frequency within the exercise prescription interact to produce health benefits. The optimal combination of these three factors is unclear, but may vary depending on the health benefit of interest (see Chapter 1). It does seem apparent from the literature, however, that with regular, moderate-intensity exercise (defined as >2 days per week, >25 min per day, at an RPE of 11–15, with no more than 2 consecutive days off), important training and health benefits can occur (see Tables 7-1 and 7-2).

This approach to exercise prescription is often called the *public health approach*. It is characterized by utilizing lowered intensity for exercise prescription, along with appropriate duration, frequency, and mode. *The use of this commonsense approach in cardiac patients will not only make the prescription itself easier to develop but will also*

TABLE 7-1. Basic principles of exercise prescription

	Minimum		Ideal	
Frequency	**3 days/week**		**4–5 days/week**	
Intensity	% peak HR 50–60	RPE 11–13	% peak HR 60–80	RPE 11–15
Duration	20 min/day		30–45 min/day	

increase patient compliance. Success is, therefore, reinforced on both sides of the equation, that is, for the physician who tries to prescribe a realistic exercise program and for the patient who attempts to comply with the prescription.

FREQUENCY AND DURATION OF EXERCISE

A more specific discussion of the basic principles of exercise prescription can be found in Chapter 3. Therefore, only general information will be presented here.

The accepted minimal frequency for both enhanced cardiovascular endurance and the general health benefits of regular exercise is 3 days per week with no more than 2 consecutive days without exercise. However, if secondary prevention of myocardial infarction and coronary artery disease progression is a goal of therapy,

TABLE 7-2. Rating of perceived exertion

6	
7	Very, very light
8	
9	Very light
10	
11	Fairly light
12	
13	Somewhat hard
14	
15	Hard
16	
17	Very hard
18	
19	Very, very hard
20	

Instructions: Ask yourself "How hard is this work?" Compare to the following: "6" is like sitting in a chair, relaxing. "20" is as hard as you have ever worked; most people have to be forced to work this hard. This is a completely subjective scale and your answer is *the right answer.*

research suggests that 1500–2000 kcal per week is the required total weekly dose of exercise[12,13] (Table 7-3). To achieve this goal, the frequency of exercise will need to be greater than 2 days per week. A person weighing 175 lb, for instance, will usually consume about 300–500 kcal per hour during moderate-intensity exercise. This means that 3 to 5 hr per week will be required to achieve the total caloric expenditure of 1500–2000 kcal per week. Most people would need 3 to 7 days per week to achieve this amount of exercise. Incidentally, caloric expenditure can be reliably estimated using simple equations and calculations, and many types of home exercise equipment display caloric expenditure automatically.[10]

The accepted minimal duration for both enhanced cardiovascular endurance and the general health benefits of regular exercise is 20 min or more per session of continuous exercise. Some reports confirm the efficacy of shorter bouts of exercise more frequently during the day.[14,15] However, for patients in whom the goal is the secondary prevention of coronary heart disease, most will require at least 20 min of exercise per session to achieve the goal of 1500–2000 kcal per week.

There are other important factors to consider when prescribing the duration of exercise, such as the patient's goals and functional limitations. For a patient whose goals include weight loss, for instance, exercise sessions should be frequent (more than 3 days per week) and relatively long in duration (more than 20 min per session) for optimal results. Additionally, patients with extremely low functional capacity or with limitations such as claudication tend to do better with frequent, short bouts of exercise. The use of this type of intermittent exercise alternating with frequent rest periods may be the only practical way to prescribe exercise for some patients.

MODE OF EXERCISE

Several modes or types of exercise can provide health benefits to patients. The ideal exercise utilizes large muscles groups in a continuous, rhythmic manner. However, for some patients, particularly those with significant functional limitations, some types of intermittent activity may be beneficial and even preferred. Walking is perhaps the most common mode utilized by the complicated as well as the uncomplicated patient because requirements for a facility, special equipment,

TABLE 7-3. Exercise prescription for secondary prevention[2,7,9,12,13]

	Amount
Frequency (days/week)	5–7
Intensity (cal/week)	1500–2000
Duration (min/day)	45–60

and specialized skills are minimal. For most people, the exercise prescription should allow for a variety of modes to prevent boredom and optimize compliance.[16]

Mode of exercise may be weight-bearing (e.g., walking, aerobics) or non–weight bearing (e.g., cycling or rowing). The choice depends on personal preference or limitations to activity imposed by other coexisting conditions such as osteoarthritis. It may also be more effective to utilize non-weight-bearing exercise (stationary cycling is excellent) for deconditioned, weak, or elderly patients during the initial sessions of an exercise program. This allows appropriate development of low levels of cardiovascular endurance and lower extremity strength/endurance conditioning in preparation for weight bearing-exercise such as walking.

Perhaps the best method for prescribing the mode of exercise should include a consideration ofboth patient preferences and physician recommendations. For example, the use of cross-country ski trainers has become extremely popular and is, in fact, a very effective method for enhancing cardiovascular endurance. This mode of exercise does require some special skills which may be difficult to learn initially. The lack of skills in utilizing this equipment may cause local muscular fatigue and an increased heart rate, and may limit the total duration and intensity of exercise. Neuromuscular fatigue and muscular endurance are often limiting factors for this type of exercise program in its initial stages. Using other forms of exercise to supplement the time necessary to develop these skills is a good approach for patients choosing this form of activity. Similar precautions should be utilized in other activities which might require the development of specific skills or specific types of muscular endurance (e.g., aerobics) prior to their use in a regular exercise program.

INTENSITY OF EXERCISE

Prescribing an appropriate intensity of exercise may be the most difficult variable in the exercise program. There are basically two ways for patients to self-monitor the intensity of their exercise program: (1) checking the heart rate during exercise with the aim of keeping it within a target heart rate range or (2) using a perceived exertion scale, which allows patients to judge the intensity of the exercise subjectively by how hard it feels to them personally. Each method has its advantages and disadvantages.

Some patient populations require the use of the heart rate for appropriate and safe monitoring of an exercise prescription. Patients who have ECG evidence of ischemia during exercise testing, even if they do not have associated angina pectoris, should have a heart rate limit during exercise which corresponds to less than 1 mm of downsloping or horizontal ST depression on the exercise test.[10] Additionally, the use of a target heart rate is critical for most patients with chronic heart failure who desire to begin an exercise program. For such patients, the target heart range is calculated most accurately from a cardiopulmonary exercise test in which oxygen consumption is measured.[17–19] Other than these reasons for limiting the exercise heart rate, there are few other reasons to limit or restrict target heart rate for cardiac patients (Table 7-4).

Some practitioners use the predicted maximum heart rate (220 − age) as a basis for developing an exercise prescription. Utilization of the predicted maximum

TABLE 7-4. Termination of exercise sessions

Signs/symptoms of Intolerance[1]
• Any sign or symptom of angina or coronary insufficiency
• Plateau or decrease in SBP, SBP > 240 mmHg or DBP > 110 mmHg
• >1 mm ST depression
• Voluntary fatigue (RPE ≥ 14–15—depending upon *your* comfort level)
• New onset or increased dysrhythmia or other ECG changes

Source: Adapted from *Guidelines for Exercise Testing and Prescription*, ed 5, American College of Sports Medicine, with permission.

heart rate, however, can introduce large errors into the exercise prescription given the wide fluctuations in patient heart rate variability and cardiopulmonary conditioning. In addition, the use of a *measured* maximum heart rate (during maximal exercise testing) can be inaccurate since many exercise tests given in a clinical situation are not truly maximal. Finally, many patients cannot take their heart rates accurately, and its use in the exercise prescription may discourage compliance.

Exercise intensity can be effectively regulated and controlled for most patients with heart disease by using the RPE[20–22] (Table 7-2). RPE has been shown to correlate with many physiologic variables that, in turn, correlate directly with the intensity of exercise.[23,24] The direct correlation of this scale with these physiologic variables allows the use of RPE to monitor exercise intensity safely and effectively. Although the use of RPE requires some training and practice, patients can learn fairly easily to use the scale in monitoring their exercise program. This allows patients to keep within limits that allow safe and effective exercise while still attaining the heart rate levels required to produce an increase in cardiovascular endurance.

The appropriate level of exertion on the RPE scale correlates with ratings of 11–15 or between "fairly light" and "hard" exertion. Teaching patients to use the scale allows them to adjust exercise on a daily basis according to a subjective feeling of wellness (how they are feeling on a given day), as well as to adjust intensity for such environmental factors as heat, wind, surface changes, or even changes in mode of exercise. RPE self-adjusts for changing conditions both internally and externally. Thus, patients can also adjust their exercise according to the conditions which directly affect exercise tolerance.

Although this method may sound somewhat foreign to both the patient and the physician, most regular exercisers regulate their daily programs by these subjective feelings. Applying a formal scale of subjective rating allows consistency from day to day, and this external tool may reassure patients of the safety of their exercise program. It also simplifies the exercise prescription for the professional because the language of such a scale is simple and understandable.

PROGRESSION OF THE EXERCISE PRESCRIPTION

The final aspect of the exercise prescription is the progression of the program toward some goal level of functional capacity. This may be determined by vocational or avocational requirements or simply by personal preference and willingness to tolerate exercise. The progression may be limited by physiologic, anatomic, or pathophysiologic factors which restrict the upper limits of exercise capacity or even the individual variables in the exercise prescription.

Progression of deconditioned patients should necessarily be slower than that of uncomplicated patients who have few limitations to the recovery process. Patients with complicated recovery may benefit from lower levels of regular physical activity/ exercise, but aggressive prescription of intensity, duration, frequency, and progression should be avoided until the underlying complications are satisfactorily resolved and treatment efficacy achieved.

Progression of intensity and duration is generally the key component of the exercise prescription which requires regular adjustment by the patient. It is generally accepted that progression of duration (distance or time) prior to progression of intensity is the preferred method. Duration can progress gradually from a minimal level initially to an ideal level several weeks later. Likewise, the progression of intensity (measured by either heart rate or RPE) from a fairly light level in the early stages of the program to a somewhat hard or even hard level after several weeks of regular exercise is an effective technique.

Although it is difficult to quantify progression, a weekly increase of 15–20% in either time or distance is appropriate until ideal levels are achieved. This would occur in about 6–8 weeks in the normal, uncomplicated cardiac patient. After achieving total duration levels equivalent to this ideal level, the intensity of exercise as regulated by RPE may be increased as indicated above.

CASE EXAMPLE

Patient History and Examination

Patient A.B. is a 50-year-old female who presented to the emergency room with chest discomfort, nausea, and diaphoresis. She was diagnosed with an evolving inferior myocardial infarction. Treatment included thrombolytic therapy and, later, successful angioplasty of a 95% right coronary artery lesion. The hospital course was uncomplicated, and A.B. was referred to the inpatient cardiac rehabilitation program. She was given a predischarge exercise test, in which she completed stage 3 of a modified Bruce protocol (approximately 4.6 METS) with a peak heart rate of 112 beats per minute and a peak blood pressure of 126/78. She completed the test without symptoms or ECG changes. A.B. was discharged with prescriptions for atenolol and aspirin. Her risk factors included hyperlipidemia, hypertension, and a sedentary lifestyle.

She reported having no regular exercise program, although she is active recreationally with boating, gardening, and yard work. She works as a manager in a sedentary job requiring minimal physical activity. She requested walking as the primary mode of exercise because of close proximity to a local walking trail and because she is "on her feet a lot."

Exercise Recommendations

Table 7-5 presents an example of the progression of an exercise program for a patient such as A.B. The prescription begins at an activity level similar to that A.B. was following at the time of hospital discharge and progresses gradually to the ideal level recommended previously. This progression is based on the assumption that there are no complications to continuing recovery and no limitations to exercise tolerance and capacity. Now in the ideal range, A.B. continues to exercise 40–45 min per day, 5 days per week. Her recovery has been uneventful, with no recurrence of symptoms and evidence of success in changing her lifestyle. Most recently, she completed stage 3 of a Bruce protocol without symptoms, ECG changes, or changes in the nuclear portion of her treadmill test.

THE USE OF INTERMITTENT EXERCISE

Intermittent exercise with periods of rest between short periods of activity is commonly used with deconditioned patients to initiate exercise programs. The basic principles of exercise prescription are utilized, except that the duration is not continuous. The prescription should progress toward the minimal levels of total duration recommended in Table 7-1. Beginning with periods of activity as short as 2–4 min, with intervening rest periods no longer than the exercise periods (ideally), will allow even very deconditioned patients to begin exercise programs with relative comfort. Initially, individualization of the rest period to accommodate patient preference is acceptable, but the patient should be encouraged to limit rest periods to the recommended length or less within four to six exercise sessions.

Progression from intermittent to continuous exercise is possible in most patients. Those with pathophysiologic limitations to exercise such as chronic heart failure, claudication, or concomitant chronic pulmonary disease may require long-term use of intermittent exercise. An example of an intermittent exercise prescription progressing to continuous exercise is presented in Table 7-6. This program may

TABLE 7-5. Progression of the exercise prescription

			Intensity	
Week	Frequency (days/week)	Duration (min)	RPE	Heart Rate (%)
1	4	20	11	50–60
2	4	24	11	50–60
3	4–5	28	11	50–60
4	4–5	32	11–13	60–75
5	5	36	11–13	60–75
6	5	40	11–13	60–75

TABLE 7-6. Intermittent exercise prescription

Week	Interval Duration (min) Exercise	Interval Duration (min) Rest	No. of Exercise Intervals	Frequency (days/week)	Total Duration (min)	Intensity (RPE)
1	4	4	3	6	12	10–11
2	6	4	3	6	18	10–11
3–4	10	4	2	5	20	11–12
5–6	15	4	2	5	30	11–12
7–8	20	5	2	4–5	40	11–13
>9	30–40	None	1	4–5	30–40	11–13

be utilized for most deconditioned, uncomplicated patients without symptoms or other factors complicating exercise tolerance.

CASE EXAMPLE

Patient History and Examination

Patient M.R., a 60-year-old male, was admitted to the hospital with a large anterior/lateral myocardial infarction. His enzyme levels, symptoms, and ECG changes confirmed the diagnosis. The hospital course was complicated, with congestive heart failure and ventricular arrhythmias. M.R. was discharged 14 days after admission. He had severe left ventricular dysfunction (EF ≈ 20%) with anterior/lateral/apical akinesis and anterior/lateral dyskinesis. He was referred to the inpatient cardiac rehabilitation program. His walking progressed to 300 ft, two times per day, at discharge without complaints or problems other than fatigue. M.R. was not given a predischarge exercise test. He was referred to the outpatient cardiac rehabilitation program for supervised exercise.

Exercise Recommendations

Table 7-7 presents an exercise prescription using intermittent exercise and rest periods throughout the first 6 weeks of the program. Note that in this case the duration progresses without progression of intensity. This enhances the ability to exercise for longer continuous periods of time. Activities of daily living, general daily activity, and vocational activity, although discontinuous in nature, generally can be paced at a level that will allow them to be completed if functional capacity supports longer periods of continuous lower-level activity. Therefore, intensity is less critical than the ability to be active for continuous periods. The exercise prescription should attempt to enhance this variable at the expense of intensity.

TABLE 7-7. Exercise prescription for patient MR

Week	Interval Duration (min) Exercise	Interval Duration (min) Rest	No. of Exercise Intervals	Total Duration (min)	Frequency (days/ week)	Intensity (RPE)
1	3	5	3	9	6	10–11
2	5	5	3	15	6	10–11
3	7	5	3	21	5	10–11
4	10	5	2	20	5	10–11
5	15	5	2	30	4–5	10–12
6	15	2–3	2	30	4–5	10–12

Note: Intensity of exercise is maintained at fairly light levels for the entire duration in order to facilitate longer duration.

PRINCIPLES OF EXERCISE PRESCRIPTION IN SPECIFIC PATIENT POPULATIONS

Most patient populations are not only amenable to exercise but also benefit from the long-term adaptations associated with regular exercise training (see Chapter 2). While the principles of exercise prescription are relatively straightforward and consistent from population to population, the contraindications and special situations are different. The professional prescribing exercise should be aware of and orient patients to these situations in the counseling session. Rather than illustrating specific exercise programs for those individuals, Table 7-8 summarizes the key factors that both the physician and the patient should be aware of and the variables that can be most effectively utilized for exercise prescription in this population.

Stable Angina

Stable angina is one of the clinical conditions most amenable to the chronic adaptations associated with chronic exercise programs. Perhaps the most beneficial adaptation to chronic exercise is an increased activity threshold for anginal symptoms. After training, symptomatic patients are able to engage in more activity (either vocational or avocational) at higher levels of energy expenditure with fewer episodes of symptoms. The mechanisms for this adaptation are well documented and quantified.[25,26]

Exercise prescriptions for patients with stable exertional angina use the same set of guidelines, with adaptation of intensity and progression. The underlying principle is to allow symptomatic patients to exercise at the upper limits of tolerance without symptoms. This may necessitate very low level exercise initially, with slower overall progression. At first, the exercise prescription should seek a level of both intensity and duration that can be achieved without symptoms and that allows a continuous duration of at least 5 min. Prophylactic nitrates are commonly utilized for symptom amelioration.

Increases in intensity and duration may be slowed by the persistence of symptoms,

TABLE 7-8. Exercise prescription for specific cardiac populations

Population	Key Factors[1]	Exercise Prescription[2]
Myocardial infarction (MI)	• Post-MI Angina • Anxiety	• RPE • SBP response to exertion • Symptoms
Post-CABG	• Incisional discomfort • Infectious processes • Anemia • New dysrhythmia (atrial fibrillation or flutter)	• RPE (11–14) • HR_{REST} + 30 BPM • Range of motion for trunk/upper extremity
Angina	• Changing pattern • Decreased exercise tolerance • Slow progression	• Symptoms • HR < ischemic HR (on GXT) • Residual fatigue minimized
Chronic heart failure	• Significant weight gain • Exertional hypotension (<rest; if able to monitor) • Abnormal exertional or resting dyspnea • Unusual or persistent fatigue after exercise	• RPE (10–13) • Exertional hypotension • Other pertinent symptoms
Dysrhythmias	• *Any* symptoms • Increasing rate or frequency	• HR < onset of dysrhythmia • Symptoms • RPE
Silent ischemia	• Associated signs or symptoms • Sudden decrease in exercise tolerance • Sudden changes in condition or overall sense of well-being (prodromal symptoms?)	• RPE preferred • If ECG changes, HR < ischemic ECG (<1.0 mm ST depression • Any other signs/symptoms
ICDs/ pacemakers	• Symptoms similar to those occurring prior to PM insertion • ICD threshold rate	• HR < ICD threshold rate • Symptoms • HR < onset dysrhythmia
Heart transplant	• HR response delayed or attenuated • Infection/rejection • Elevated HR_{REST}	• RPE • Signs/symptoms
Valvular heart disease	• Symptoms associated with intolerance • Fatigue	• RPE • HR < onset symptoms • Duration/intensity < onset extreme fatigue

Source: Adapted from *Guidelines for Exercise Testing and Prescription,* ed 5, American College of Sports Medicine, with permission

[1]Those factors which should be specifically covered in precautions by the exercise counselor.

[2]Those variables which should be utilized to control the intensity of exercise.

necessitating smaller changes in the progression. See Table 7-7 for a slower progression that may be similar to the one utilized with symptomatic patients. Generally, progression in duration is preferable to progression in intensity until continuous activity of 10–15 min is possible. At that point in the program, increases in intensity may be more easily accomplished. Appropriate exercise testing in patients with exertional angina allows one to establish a peak exercise heart rate for the exercise prescription (see Chapter 5).

Symptomatic patients, particularly those with low functional capacity, benefit from referral to outpatient cardiac rehabilitation units initially, not only because of the guidance and monitoring they offer but also because of the support available in those settings and because of the associated health benefits of such programs (see Chapter 1). The slowness of the progress for patients with low functional capacity is often disappointing to them and may affect their adherence in the short term.

Chronic Heart Failure

Patients with severe left ventricular dysfunction and chronic heart failure (CHF) have often been advised to limit their activity and regular exercise. More recent findings indicate that these patients can benefit from a regular exercise program and can exercise safely. Specifically, CHF patients exhibit skeletal muscle changes that decrease their tolerance to activity. It has been shown that these effects can be reversed and skeletal muscle function improved by regular exercise.[18,19]

Prescribing exercise for patients with severe left ventricular dysfunction and CHF is similar to prescribing for other populations that are deconditioned and may not tolerate continuous exercise. Refer to Table 7-8 for the key factors and variables which should be utilized as the basis of the exercise prescription. This patient population can benefit from early referral to a supervised, monitored outpatient cardiac rehabilitation program. Table 7-7 illustrates a typical exercise progression for a CHF patient (M.R., discussed above).

Exercise prescription, especially in the most deconditioned CHF patients, is best done using intermittent exercise. The rate of progression may be altered, depending on the initial level of functional capacity and the tolerance for continuous exercise. Often the most deconditioned patients tolerate continuous exercise of longer duration poorly and are maintained on a program utilizing intermittent periods of exercise indefinitely. The program can be further abbreviated with respect to continuous duration by eliminating previous steps in the progression. *One of the most significant factors indicating intolerance to exercise is abnormal, prolonged fatigue in the postexercise period. If this symptom develops, it may indicate that the intermittent bouts are too long or that the rest period is too short.*

CHF patients are another group of patients who may derive significant benefits from enrollment in an outpatient cardiac rehabilitation program. Supervision and guidance, especially in the initial period of regular exercise, may assist the physician in clarifying symptoms, preventing acute bouts of CHF, and structuring proper, safe progression of the exercise program. Support and reinforcement, particularly from the primary care physician, are also important for exercise adherence in this population.

Post–Coronary Artery Bypass Surgery

CASE EXAMPLE

Patient History and Examination

Patient M.L. was admitted to the hospital for coronary artery bypass surgery after a positive exercise thallium test and an angiogram showing two-vessel coronary artery disease in the left anterior descending, obtuse marginal, and circumflex arteries. He completed the hospital course without complications and was discharged on postoperative day 5. He had been walking approximately .75 mile per day without problems or symptoms. He was not given a predischarge treadmill test.

Exercise Recommendations

The exercise prescription for M.L. is relatively straightforward and, barring posthospital complications, he will, like most uncomplicated post-CABS patients, progress quickly. Early postoperative fatigue may require initial use of intermittent exercise for tolerance, but after 3 to 4 weeks many CABS patients progress on intermittent programs more quickly or can switch to continuous exercise. Some combination of the programs illustrated in Tables 7-6 and 7-7 may be applicable. Refer to Table 7-8 for "key factors" and an exercise prescription for these patients.

Dysrhythmias

The diverse, complicated population of dysrhythmia patients makes generalization of exercise principles difficult. Perhaps the key factors in tolerance of exercise are medical control of the altered rhythm and patient tolerance of the dysrhythmia itself. Exercise is not necessarily contraindicated in these patients, but careful attention to any changes in the dysrhythmia, any association with increasing exercise intensity or duration, or any changes in clinical status are important to patient safety.[10,25,26] For these reasons, it is often important to use monitored, supervised exercise in this population.

Patients with good control and tolerance of the dysrhythmia, those with pacemakers or implantable cardio-defibrillators (ICDs) and those without rate-related dysrhythmias should tolerate a moderate exercise program such as the one illustrated in Table 7-5. It may be necessary to modify the program for complicating conditions such as CHF, left ventricular dysfunction, lower tolerance of the dysrhythmia or of pharmacologic therapy, or other complicating factors.

Valvular Heart Disease

Valvular heart disease, with repair and subsequent improvement in functional capacity and clinical status, does not preclude exercise. In many cases, patients will benefit from the conditioning that regular exercise offers and tolerate moderate exercise well. Their response may be little different from that of the normal population, and an exercise prescription similar to post-CABG patients (see the case of M.L. above) is advisable.

Patients without repair and who remain symptomatic may be more difficult. Attention to complicating conditions such as dysrhythmias, CHF, of even extreme fatigue may make an exercise regimen difficult to tolerate and an exercise prescription difficult (see Chapter 6). Intermittent exercise is often required for the best results. See Table 7-8 for factors and exercise prescription information. This group benefits from referral to a monitored outpatient cardiac rehabilitation program.

Hypertension

Hypertension has been shown to be amenable to regular endurance exercise, and many patients attain improved blood pressure control with a regular program of moderate exercise. The recommendations of the 26th Bethesda conference[27] state that the presence of mild (systolic blood pressure [SBP] = 140–159 mm Hg; diastolic blood pressure [DBP] = 90–99 mm Hg) or moderate (SBP = 160–179 mm Hg; DBP = 100–109 mm Hg) hypertension, without evidence of target organ damage or coexistent heart disease, should not limit participation in sports. The presence of severe hypertension (SBP ≥ 180 mm Hg; DBP ≥ 110 mm Hg) requires that the athlete not participate in sports that require a high muscular force with little change in muscle length or joint movement (i.e., static exercise) until the blood pressure is controlled.

Although the direct evidence that essential hypertension is affected by adaptations to exercise remains controversial, there is little question that the epidemiologic evidence calls for regular exercise as an intervention. In fact, regular, low- to moderate-intensity exercise has been shown to be very helpful in controlling mild hypertension.[28–31] The most effective combination of intensity, duration, and frequency is not precisely known, but it appears that an exercise program of low to moderate intensity and duration is at least as safe and effective as a higher-intensity program. Table 7-5 presents a typical progression for patients with essential hypertension without concomitant complicating factors.

Syncope

Syncope is a common symptom among the general population, affecting approximately 5% of the elderly population and up to 15% of young adults; it may be even more common among patients with cardiovascular disease.[32,33] A patient with syncope should be prohibited from performing exercise until the etiology of the syncope has been identified. In at least a third of cases, a detailed patient history and physical examination can identify the cause of syncope.[34] Causes of syncope can be grouped into four main categories:

1. *Cardiac* (mechanical and/or electrical cardiac dysfunction).
2. *Vascular* (e.g., vasovagal or hypersensitive carotid sinus).
3. *Noncardiovascular* (e.g., seizure, metabolic disorders, or drug use).

4. *Unexplained* (up to 50% of cases are unexplained even after specialized testing).

Cardiac syncope is the most worrisome cause of syncope, with a 1-year mortality rate of 20–30%. Noncardiovascular syncope carries a lower but still substantial 1-year mortality rate of 10–15%. Vascular syncope and unexplained syncope are associated with 1-year mortality rates of approximately 5% or less.[35,36]

Specialized testing can help identify and quantify the cause of syncope in many cases. Ambulatory electrocardiographic event monitors, for example, can be helpful when dysrhythmias are the cause of syncope. Electrophysiologic testing may be required in some instances, both to identify the dysrhythmia and to monitor the response to therapy. Tilt table testing may help identify patients with vasovagal syncope and can be used to monitor the response to therapy. Unfortunately, the specificity of the test is somewhat limited.[37]

If correctable causes of syncope are identified and treated, patients can be advised with caution to begin physical activity. Vasovagal syncope is relatively common in highly trained athletes and can often be controlled with pharmacologic therapy.[38] Many patients with nonrecurrent, unexplained syncope can participate in exercise activities but should be monitored closely for recurrent symptoms. Clearly, exercise activities should be prohibited in patients with cardiac or noncardiovascular syncope in whom the cause of the syncope cannot be controlled and in patients with recurrent syncope of any etiology. Once patients are cleared for physical activity, they should initially avoid activities that would be potentially dangerous if the syncope recurs (bicycling, mountain climbing, etc.) until it is clear that the cause of the syncope has been well controlled and the syncope does not recur.

THE EFFECT OF CARDIOVASCULAR DRUGS ON PATIENT EVALUATION AND THE EXERCISE PRESCRIPTION

Since many patients with cardiovascular diseases or those at high risk require treatment with cardioactive drugs, it is important to consider the potential impact of such drugs on the preparticipation evaluation and the exercise prescription.[39,40] The following drugs are of particular importance.

Beta-Blocking Agents

Since beta-blocking agents can significantly reduce resting and peak heart rates, their use makes reliance on heart rate in exercise testing and in monitoring exercise intensity somewhat problematic. Few patients on beta blockers are able to attain a peak exercise heart rate during a maximal exercise test which meets the traditional definition for a truly maximal test, i.e., at least 85% of the predicted maximal heart rate for age. The predicted maximal heart rate for a patient taking a beta-blocking agent is approximately 10–20% less than that predicted by the traditional definition (220 − age). In general, the higher the patient's heart rate prior to beta-blocker therapy, the greater the decrease in heart rate after initiation of therapy. In addition, the type of beta blocker will influence the heart rate effect; agents with intrinsic sympathomimetic activity (ISA) will have less of an impact on heart rate than agents without ISA.

The modified predicted maximal heart rate for a patient with a high normal resting heart rate and on a non-ISA beta blocker, for instance, could be estimated as (.80)(220 − age). For a patient with a low normal resting heart rate who is taking a beta blocker with ISA, the modified formula for estimating maximal heart rate would be (.90)(220 − age). Practically speaking, these adjustments are most important in patients who do *not* undergo a maximal exercise test prior to initiating their exercise program yet want to monitor exercise intensity by heart rate. For example, if such a patient wishes to exercise at 65% of the predicted maximal heart rate, the prescription should be changed so that the goal is 65% of the modified predicted maximal heart rate described above. To simplify the exercise prescription for such patients, the RPE scale discussed earlier in this chapter can be used to guide the patient's exercise intensity.

In patients with known heart disease who are on beta-blocker therapy and who require close monitoring of their heart rate during exercise, the maximal heart rate should be *measured* during maximal exercise testing rather than estimated by the patient's age alone. In this manner, the usual methods of calculating exercise target heart rates (heart rate reserve method, for example) can be accurately used.

In addition, the accuracy of exercise electrocardiography is somewhat hampered by beta-blocker usage. Beta blockers decrease myocardial oxygen demand by decreasing the blood pressure and heart rate and may actually prevent or delay the onset of exertional ischemia in patients during exercise testing. The decision to continue or discontinue beta-blocker therapy prior to exercise testing largely depends on the purpose of the exercise test. In the patient with atypical exertional chest pain who undergoes exercise testing for *diagnostic* purposes, beta-blocker therapy may need to be tapered during the week or two prior to testing. By contrast, in the patient with known coronary artery disease who is undergoing exercise testing for *exercise prescription* purposes, beta blockers need not be discontinued prior to testing. In fact, in such patients, it is usually important that the test be performed while the patient is on the same dose of beta blocker used during exercise training.

There are several potential drawbacks to beta-blocker therapy for the patient-athlete. First, beta blockers may blunt maximal exercise tolerance, although it appears that they do not significantly blunt the exercise training effect.[41] In the patient with exertional angina, exercise tolerance may actually increase on beta-blocker therapy. This is due to the fact that patients are able to perform a given amount of work at lower heart rate and blood pressure levels, effectively raising the "ischemic threshold." Many patients on beta blockers note significant fatigue, probably due to cardiovascular as well as metabolic side effects (altered fatty acid and glycogen metabolism). Finally, patients who participate as competitive athletes in events that require steadiness of hand (riflery, archery, etc.) should be aware that the use of beta blockers is banned in such sports by several athletic governing bodies (e.g., the International Olympic Committee and the NCAA).[42]

Nitrates

Use of nitrates is common among patients with coronary artery disease and can significantly enhance angina-free exercise tolerance by increasing myocardial oxygen supply and decreasing myocardial oxygen demand. Nitrates have little or no effect on exercise tolerance in patients who are free from inducible myocardial ischemia. Like beta blockers, nitrates can prevent or delay the onset of inducible ischemia during maximal exercise testing, leading to false-negative results. When exercise testing is performed for *diagnostic* purposes, nitrates may need to be discontinued temporarily. Nitrates reduce resting and exercise blood pressure slightly and lead to a mild reflex tachycardia, but these changes generally have little or no effect on the exercise prescription for most patients.

Since nitrates are usually administered intermittently to prevent tolerance (i.e., patients usually have a nitrate-free window each day), it is important that patients plan their exercise regimens so that they occur during active nitrate treatment periods. Some patients may prefer to administer a short-acting nitrate just prior to exercise to prevent exertional ischemia. This, however, may provoke hypotension and even syncope in some patients and should only be initiated under close monitoring by a medical professional.

Calcium-Channel Antagonists

Calcium-channel antagonists are widely used as antihypertensive drugs. They can produce significant improvement in exercise capacity in patients with inducible myocardial ischemia by increasing the threshold for myocardial ischemia. Like beta blockers and nitrates, calcium-channel antagonists may need to be discontinued temporarily in patients undergoing an exercise test for *diagnostic* purposes. Nifedipine reduces blood pressure and often leads to a reflex tachycardia. Diltiazem and verapamil, on the other hand, have effects more similar to those of beta blockers, reducing blood pressure and heart rate, both at rest and with exercise. In general, these effects invalidate the usual age-predicted estimations of maximal heart rate, but as explained in the discussion of beta blockers above, such effects have little practical importance for most patient-athletes with cardiovascular disease. Patients who require heart rate monitoring during exercise should usually undergo exercise testing while on the dose of calcium-channel antagonist that they will use during exercise training.

Digitalis

Digitalis appears to increase exercise tolerance in two subsets of patients: those with either atrial fibrillation or chronic heart failure. No alterations need to be made in the exercise prescription for patients on digitalis therapy other than those dictated by their underlying condition (i.e., atrial fibrillation or chronic heart failure). Digitalis, however, may produce sagging of the ST segment, which can be difficult to differentiate from ischemia-induced ST depression. For this reason, digitalis should ideally be discontinued approximately 2 weeks prior to exercise testing for *diagnostic* purposes.

Other Medications

Quinidine has been found to produce false-negative exercise test results in some people. Procainamide, by contrast, has been reported to produce false-positive exercise test results. Diuretics may produce hypokalemia and false-positive exercise test results. Their use is generally banned by many athletic governing bodies (e.g., the International Olympic Committee).[42] Nicotine may increase blood pressure and heart rate, which can *decrease* the ischemic threshold in some patients. As a result, exercise tolerance may be decreased in patients with inducible ischemia.

SUMMARY

1. Most patients with cardiovascular disease can exercise safely and attain significant health benefits. It appears that a ideal level of physical activity that would help optimize the health of persons with cardiovascular disease is approximately 1500–2000 kcal.
2. Many patients with cardiovascular disease benefit from an exercise program that begins with relatively low-intensity, short exercise sessions 2–3 days per week. Intermittent exercise (the use of multiple short bouts of exercise alternating with brief rest periods) may be particularly useful in patients with significant functional limitations.
3. Exercise sessions can be gradually advanced to an idea level or "dose" by increasing the duration of exercise first, followed by appropriate increases in the frequency and intensity of exercise. The focus of exercise sessions for most patients should be on the duration and frequency of exercise, with the goal of improving endurance for activities of daily living.
4. Supervised cardiac rehabilitation programs are important for higher-risk individuals or those with significantly impaired functional capacity. Some lower-risk patients may also benefit from such programs, especially if they need structured support to maintain an exercise program.
5. Several cardioactive drugs may affect the accuracy of the exercise test. In persons who use heart rate to monitor their exercise intensity, the use of some drugs may necessitate alterations in the target heart rates specified in their exercise prescription. When exercise testing is performed for *diagnostic* purposes, cardioactive drugs may need to be temporarily discontinued to maximize the accuracy of the test.

REFERENCES

1. Gordon NF, Kohl HW III, Blair SN: Life style exercise: A new strategy to promote physical activity for adults, *J Cardiopulm Rehabil* 13:161–163, 1993.
2. Blair SN: Physical fitness and all-cause mortality: A prospective study of healthy men and women, *JAMA* 262(17):2395–2401, 1989.
3. Blair SN: Exercise and health. In *Sports Science Exchange*, Vol. 3, No. 29, Chicago, Gatorade Science Institute, 1990.

4. Caspersen CJ, Christenson GM, Pollard RA: Status of the 1990 physical fitness and exercise objectives—evidence from NHIS 1985, *Public Health Rep* 101:587–592, 1986.
5. Duncan J, Gordon NF, Scott CB: Women walking for health and fitness: How much is enough? *JAMA* 266(23):3295–3299, 1991.
6. Koplan JP, Caspersen CJ, Powell K: Physical activity, physical fitness and health: Time to act. *JAMA* 262:2437, 1989.
7. Paffenbarger RS, Jr, Hyde RT, Wing AL, et al: Physical activity and all-cause mortality and longevity of college alumni. *N Engl J Med* 314:605–613, 1986.
8. Posner JD, Gorman KM, Windsor-Landsberg L, et al: Low to moderate intensity endurance training in healthy older adults: Physiological responses after four months. *J Am Geriatr Soc* 40:1–7, 1992.
9. Powell KE, Thompson PD, Caspersen CJ, et al: Physical activity and the incidence of coronary heart disease. *Ann Rev Public Health* 8:253–287, 1987.
10. American College of Sports Medicine: *Guidelines for Exercise Testing and Prescription*, ed 4. Philadelphia, Lea and Febiger, 1991.
11. Pollock ML: The quantification of endurance training programs. Wilmore JH (ed): In *Exercise and Sport Sciences Reviews*. New York, Academic Press, 1973, pp 155–188.
12. Hambrecht R, Niebauer J, Marburger C, et al: Various intensities of leisure time physical activity in patients with coronary artery disease: Effects on cardiorespiratory fitness and progression of coronary atherosclerotic lesions. *J Am Coll Cardiol* 22:468–477, 1993.
13. Paffenbarger RS Jr, Hale WE: Work activity and coronary heart mortality. *N Engl J Med* 292:545–550, 1975.
14. DeBusk RF, Stenestrand U, Sheehan M, et al: Training effects of long versus short bouts of exercise in healthy subjects. *Am J Cardiol* 65:1010–1013, 1990.
15. DeBusk RF, Haskell WL: Do multiple short bouts of exercise really produce the same benefits as single long bouts? (Reply to a letter to the editor). *Am J Cardiol* 67:325–326, 1991.
16. King AC, Martin JE: Exercise adherence and maintenance. In J. Larry Durstine, et al. (eds.) *Resource Manual for Exercise Testing and Prescription*, ed 2. Philadelphia, Lea and Febiger, 1993, pp 443–454.
17. Davies SW, Emery TM, Watling MIL, et al: A critical threshold of exercise capacity in the ventilatory response to exercise in heart failure. *Br Heart J* 65:179–183, 1991.
18. Sullivan M, Higginbotham MB, and Cobb FR: Exercise training in patients with chronic heart failure delays ventilatory anaerobic threshold and improves submaximum exercise performance. *Circulation* 79:324–329, 1989.
19. Sullivan MJ, and Cobb FR: The anaerobic threshold in chronic heart failure. *Circulation* 81(Suppl II):II-47–II-58, 1990.
20. Ceci R, and Hassmen P: Self-monitored exercise at three different RPE intensities in treadmill vs. field running. *Med Sci Sports Exerc* 23:732–738, 1991.
21. Bayles CM, Metz KF, Robertson R, et al: Perceptual regulation of prescribed exercise. *J Cardiopulm Rehabil* 10:25–31, 1990.
22. Spelman CC, Pate RR, Macera CA, et al: Self-selected exercise intensity of habitual walkers. *Med Sci Sports Exerc* 25:1174–1179, 1993.
23. Noble BJ: Clinical applications of perceived exertion. *Med Sci Sports Exerc* 14:406–411, 1982.
24. Pandolf KB: Advances in the study and application of perceived exertion. *Sport Sci Rev* 11:118–158, 1983.
25. Wenger NK, Hellerstein H: *Rehabilitation of the Coronary Patient*, ed 3. New York, Churchill Livingstone, 1992, p 371.
26. Leon AS: Position paper of the American Association of Cardiovascular and Pulmonary

Rehabilitation. Scientific evidence of the value of cardiac rehabilitation services with emphasis on patients following myocardial infarction. I. Exercise conditioning component. *J Cardiopulm Rehabil* 10:79–87, 1990.
27. Maron BJ, Mitchell JH: 26th Bethesda Conference: Recommendations for determining eligibility for competition in athletes with cardiovascular abnormalities. *J Am Coll Cardiol* 24:845–899, 1994.
28. Gordon NF, Scott CB, Wilkinson WJ, et al: Exercise and mild essential hypertension recommendations for adults. *Sports Med* 10:390–404, 1990.
29. Paffenbarger RS Jr, Jung DL, Leung W, et al: Physical activity and hypertension: An epidemiological view. *Ann Med* 23:319–327, 1991.
30. Tipton CM; Exercise, training and hypertension. In *ACSM Series Exerc Sports Sci Rev* 19:447–505, 1991.
31. American College of Sports Medicine Position Stand: Physical activity, physical fitness and hypertension. *Med Sci Sp Exerc* 25:i–x, 1993.
32. Whiteside-Yim C: Syncope in the elderly: A clinical approach. *Geriatrics* 42:37–41, 1987.
33. Boudoulas H, Weissler AM, Lewis RP, et al: The clinical diagnosis of syncope. *Curr Probl Cardiol* 7:1–40, 1982.
34. Kapoor WN: Evaluation and management of the patient with syncope. *JAMA* 268:2553–2560, 1992.
35. Kapoor WN, Karpf M, Wieand S, et al: A prospective evaluation and follow-up of patients with syncope. *N Engl J Med* 309:197–204, 1983.
36. Day SC, Cook EF, Funkenstein H, et al: Evaluation and outcome of emergency room patients with transient loss of consciousness. *Am J Med* 73:15–23, 1982.
37. Zipes DP, Garson A: 26th Bethesda Conference: Task Force 6: Arrhythmias. *J Am Coll Cardiol* 24:S276–S283, 1994.
38. Calkins H, Seifert M, Morady F: Clinical presentation and long-term follow-up of athletes with exercise-induced vasodepressor syncope. *Am Heart J* 129:1159–1164, 1995.
39. Van Camp SP: Pharmacologic factors in exercise and exercise testing. In Blair SN, Painter P, Pate RR, et al (eds): *Resource Manual for Guidelines for Exercise Testing and Prescription*. American College of Sports Medicine. Philadelphia, Lea and Febiger, 1988, pp 135–152.
40. Wenger NK: Cardiovascular drugs: Effects on exercise testing and exercise training of the coronary patient. In Wenger NK (ed): *Exercise and the Heart*. Philadelphia, FA Davis, 1985, pp 133–143.
41. Horgan JH, Teo KK: Training response in patients with coronary artery disease receiving beta-adrenergic blocking drugs with or without partial agonist activity. *J Cardiovasc Pharm* 5:1019–1024, 1983.
42. Wadler GI, Hainline B: *Drugs and the Athlete*. Philadelphia, FA Davis, 1989.

♦ CHAPTER EIGHT ♦

LEGAL ASPECTS OF EXERCISE IN PERSONS WITH CARDIOVASCULAR DISORDERS

William G. Herbert, Ph.D., FACSM
David L. Herbert, J.D.

INTRODUCTION

This chapter addresses legal considerations that affect physicians who render eligibility decisions for sports participation by individuals who have suspected or diagnosed circulatory disorders. Emphasis is given to issues surrounding decisions on clearance for sports activities and competitions that are known to impose near-maximal cardiovascular stress in the setting of organized competition. Cases are discussed in some sections to help illustrate the various ways in which legal issues may complicate the process. Explicit suggestions are made whereby physicians may approach these decisions so as to limit their legal exposure, and do so without compromising the integrity of the physician–patient relationship that has been a hallmark of the medical profession since the days of Hippocrates some 2000 years ago.[1] The information presented here is no substitute for the individualized legal advice which every practitioner must secure in support of his or her clinical practice.

CASE EXAMPLE

A 19-year-old boy who is an outstanding player for a local university's basketball team sees you following a fainting episode he suffered while running sprints at the end of a practice session. He had two syncopal episodes when he was in high school but did not report them to anyone and did not have them evaluated. He has been told that he has a murmur but that it is an "innocent" murmur.

What are the legal implications for you, the primary care physician, in assessing this patient's fitness to participate in athletic competition? If you uncover a health condition that could be potentially life-threatening, are you obligated to inform the university officials, even without the patient's consent? If you recommend that the patient not be allowed to participate on the university's team due to a high-risk medical condition, are you liable for the patient's potential loss of future income (i.e., from playing professional basketball)?

SCOPE OF THE PROBLEM

Experience has shown that participation in physically challenging sports activity carries certain risks of harm, even for those who are considered to be healthy. Public perception regards these risks as so low that they almost escape the collective consciousness until national media draw attention to such tragedies, as occurred with the sudden death of Hank Gathers.[2] Epidemiologists and health care professionals perceive the actual risks more clearly and have compiled observations that allow some characterization of the cardiovascular risks (e.g., fewer than 7 deaths/ 1,000,000 athletes/year among younger amateur adult contestants).[3] Using these meager retrospective mortality data along with a sports classification schema, it is possible to create a simple framework for clinical decision making. This approach applies risk stratification criteria to allow a rational evaluation of the athlete with a cardiovascular disorder against a backdrop of factors such as cardiac demand, bodily collision potential, and environmental hazards of the contest.[4] While this framework seems quite reasonable, the paucity of medical data may leave physicians uncomfortable in deciding simply to disqualify or substantially limit a patient's activities when the patient is highly motivated to participate, very unlikely to harm others, and willing to accept the risks.[5]

A Dilemma for Physicians

When confronted with responsibilities to examine and evaluate an individual with cardiovascular disorders for competition, the physician is sometimes faced with unreasonable expectations from athletes, their families, and other interested parties who may ascribe enormous importance to being cleared for competition. Physicians with direct involvement in such matters have commented on these difficulties, emphasizing that the pressures grow in proportion to the level of competition, the talent and celebrity of the athlete, and the material rewards involved.[2,6] In addition, the team physician in a prestigious position with a high-profile athletic program is sometimes faced with conflicts of interest in these situations, making it unclear whether the welfare of the patient is always paramount.[7,8]

These circumstances challenge the physician ethically, complicate the physician–patient relationship, and may expose the physician to substantial legal risks. Public consciousness comes quickly to the forefront whenever serious injury or death strikes a celebrated athlete during a major sports event. Invariably, questions follow in an effort to understand the cause(s); second guess any professional judgments that may have placed the athlete in harm's way; and, more often than not, seek to fix responsibility for the tragedy. In the case of athletes who are suspected or known to have cardiovascular disorders and then die in the course of training or competition, as with the tragic deaths of Hank Gathers[9] and Reggie Lewis,[10] many interested parties look to the sports medicine physician for answers.

In contrast, the physician may exercise medical judgment and conclude that the risks are sufficient to prohibit participation or delay requalification of a particular individual for a sports activity. Then, paradoxically, pressures from athletes and/or third parties, as well as legal challenges, may occur in efforts to override the decision so that the athlete can compete despite acknowledgment of the risks.[11]

IMPLICATIONS OF THE LEGAL SYSTEM

Duties of Licensed Physicians

DEFINITIONS IN STATE STATUTES

State statutes governing the practice of medicine generally provide that only licensed physicians have the legal authority to evaluate, diagnose, and treat individuals for the purposes of relieving pain, reducing physical impairment, and restoring health, whether such activities are performed within the context of sports or not.[12] Consequently, if questions are raised regarding the actions of a physician in examining, screening, and clearing a patient-athlete with a cardiovascular disorder, there is a clear legal expectation for the sports medicine practitioner(s) to discharge their services in a manner consistent with protecting the individual from harmful consequences. This same expectation very likely would extend to any and all licensed and nonlicensed sports medicine providers who are specifically involved in providing services related to the clearance or exercise limitations imposed on the patient-athlete in question. These state statutes typically are written to give broad authority to physicians and specific, limited practice authorizations for other licensed allied health care providers.[13] For these reasons, all providers in sports medicine, particularly the primary physician, should recognize that it is legally risky to delegate authority to other members of the sports medicine team in medical matters that are potentially life-threatening. Likewise, in these areas of such crucial importance to the athlete's health, nonphysician providers (e.g., athletic trainers, physical therapists, and exercise physiologists) should not act independently or in lieu of a decision by the physician in charge. To do so would carry risk of both civil and criminal charges related to the unauthorized practice of medicine.[12]

SPECIALIZED PHYSICIAN CREDENTIALS

Separate statutory authority per se is not available in the area of sports medicine, let alone in the more narrow specialization of sports cardiology. Very recently, however, the American Board of Medical Specialties created subspecialty certifications for physicians in sports medicine.[14] Physicians who are involved in clearing athletes with cardiovascular disorders, acting in either a primary or a consulting capacity, might someday expect to be defendants in malpractice claims. In such legal challenges, it is almost always the case that questions arise about the physician's special qualifications to render such medical decisions. Medical board certification in internal medicine or cardiology helps to provide presumptive evidence of qualification, and now, so does board certification in sports medicine.[13] Additional certifications are available from other physician associations. These special certifications and credentials, if relevant and maintained as current, in general may demonstrate access to special knowledge and peer recognition of competence. Physicians engaged in these cardiovascular clearance decisions should secure such credentials, not only to reduce their legal risks but also to maintain current knowledge and skills through the activities required in the qualifying process.

FACTORS AFFECTING THE SCOPE OF THE PHYSICIAN'S LEGAL DUTY

Physicians may act professionally in a variety of contexts relative to these medical screening procedures. Consequently, their relationship to the patient and to any third parties will affect the scope of their legal duty to the patient-athlete. Hence, there may be somewhat different legal expectations for the personal physician conducting screenings for his or her patient, the team physician who serves as a volunteer or paid employee, the specialist acting as a consultant in performing special medical assessments, or even the physician who is retained to offer a second opinion at the request of the athlete-patient.

In instances where the physician is retained by a club, facility, team, school, university, or similar entity, the duty owed to the patient may be limited to conducting the required medical services and rendering judgments in a reasonable manner. Two different contemporary court cases support this interpretation of a more limited physician–patient relationship in such circumstances.[11] In both *Sitomer v. Half Hollow Hills Central School District* (1987) and *Colombo v. Sewanhaka Central High School District No. 2* (1976), medical evaluation of high school students led to their exclusion from participation when the medical officers of the school systems had judged that participation might constitute a danger to these students. Suits were brought against the schools and physicians by the students and parents on the basis of multiple claims. The courts dismissed both cases, finding that the schools and their medical officers should be free to apply reasonable judgments in the course of screening students for participation in athletic programs.

In the case of *Colombo v. Sewanhaka Central High School District*, the court also upheld the school and its physician, even though the student and his parents were willing to assume the risks of injury and indemnify the school board against any damages arising from untoward events.[11]

The Question of Immunity

With heightened awareness of the diagnostic and legal difficulties surrounding these clearance issues, some practitioners hope to see revisions of state laws that would grant them some immunity from claims and suits. Generally, such immunity has been available in many states, but only for the physician who donates services to the team, and even this protection typically has been restricted to the provision of emergency medical treatment. Current statutes in some states, such as Ohio and Maryland, seem to provide a possible basis for the *legal argument* that the preparticipation medical exam and decisions flowing therefrom should be encompassed in the services of the physician volunteer for which legal immunity may be provided (in Maryland, s 5-309.4: Liability of volunteer sports program physicians).[15]

Confidentiality, Disclosure, and Minors

Maron has commented on the legal quandary sometimes faced by physicians who conduct screening examinations with patient-athletes who are minors.[5] The problem often arises when a medical cause is found to exclude the minor from competition. Upon citing physician–patient confidentiality requirements, the legally responsible family member (usually a parent) may request that the physician not disclose relevant medical findings to the school or team officials who control access to competition. This problem can also arise with the patient who is a legally competent adult, but it can be more complicated in the case of a minor. Depending on the sport, failure to disclose the medical finding may put the patient and perhaps others at risk of serious harm (e.g., in downhill ski competition). Maron's speculation on this seems entirely reasonable, i.e., that the law would be most reluctant to impose a disclosure obligation on physicians that is contrary to medical ethics or professional responsibilities. There are no simple solutions to this problem. In certain cases, the physician may feel compelled to disclose relevant information on weighing the relative risks of participation to the patient against the obligation to protect others in the community who might suffer harm as a consequence of the patient's participation.

Standards of Care

LEGAL CONTEXT

The health care profession as a whole has moved toward the development and promulgation of written standards of practice for utilization by those rendering care.[16] To date, an estimated 30,000 documents have been disseminated that may have implications for the legal standards of care in the health care field. As many as 100 of these may have specific implications for the practice of sports medicine![17] While this situation may signal concern and resistance by some practitioners, utilization of relevant standards in the delivery of health care is a professional expectation, and adherence is often critical to a defense against claims of malpractice. In reality, and unfortunately, the current experience of attorneys involved in malpractice litigation suggests that deviation from practice guidelines is cited nearly twice as often by plaintiffs in malpractice claims against physicians as is adherence to guidelines by defense attorneys.[18] Failure to meet the appropriate standard in the delivery of care to a patient may contribute to demonstration of a proximate cause of harm to that patient and, therefore, may be legally actionable.

SPORTS MEDICINE PRACTICE GUIDELINES AND RECOMMENDATIONS

The physician's conduct in evaluating and clearing patient-athletes with cardiovascular disorders may be judged by the courts in reference to consensus guidelines from the medical field, testimony of expert witnesses, and reference to state statutes that define the legal authority for medical practice. Guidelines developed by medical, scientific, and allied health organizations that may affect interpretation of the standard of care in sports medicine include, but are not limited to, those issued by the American College of Sports Medicine,[19] the American College of Cardiology with the American Heart Association,[20] the National Collegiate Athletic Association,[21] and the American Academy of Pediatrics.[22] Some of these guidelines-type documents provide specific recommendations regarding medical indications for exercise testing, interpretation of function and fitness in the context of exercise evaluation, and exercise prescription.[19,20] If utilized appropriately to guide individual medical judgments, these highly authoritative standards-type documents have the potential to raise the overall quality of medical care.

THE 26TH BETHESDA CONFERENCE RECOMMENDATIONS

The recommendations of the recent 26th Bethesda Conference on eligibility for competition in athletes with cardiovascular abnormalities represents a landmark contribution that may help physicians resolve many of these difficult clinical decisions.[23] The Bethesda recommendations undoubtedly will find their way into the malpractice litigation when questions arise as to the standard of care. Readers will find three excellent articles in the publication that provide a valuable perspective on the ethical and medicolegal considerations in eligibility decisions affecting athletes with identified cardiovascular disorders.[5,24,25] Inspection of the six Task Force Reports reveals a certain consistency in format and presentation that should reduce ambiguity of application. Whether the Report addresses congenital heart disease or arrhythmias, there seems to be clarity on the clinical definition of the abnormality, what laboratory measures might be needed to confirm a diagnosis, and what functional criteria are needed to grade the disorder for clinical severity. Throughout the six Reports are explicit recommendations concerning the types of competitive sports in which the athlete might participate without restriction, with certain restrictions, or with none at all. In some sections, circumstances also are described wherein participation is indicated only after evaluation of exercise test results and development of a specific exercise prescription.[26] All in all, these Reports reach a level of exactness that can be very helpful to the physician who seeks to make judgments in a great variety of cases involving cardiovascular abnormalities. The legal risks attendant on any malpractice claim and suit may be reduced by following protocols that are consistent with the contents of these Reports or by carefully documenting in clinical records the individual medical considerations that may justify deviation therefrom.

Implications of Federal and State Statutes

Federal laws, including the Americans with Disabilities Act of 1990 and the Rehabilitation Act of 1973, as well as similarly focused state statutes, prohibit unjustified discrimination against athletes with physical impairments amounting to protected disabilities or handicaps. Essentially, these laws provide that an impaired athlete is entitled to the same opportunities to compete as others, so long as the individual's risk of harm to self and others is not reasonably at issue and the team or sponsors are able to conduct a safe program. Mitten[25] has described a relevant case, *Larkin v. Archdiocese of Cincinnati*, in which a high school football player was prohibited from playing due to a medical judgment based on the diagnosis of structural heart disease. His parents were willing to waive future claims against the school if he was allowed to compete. The court did not find reason to support the parents' claim of arbitrary discrimination based on the Rehabilitation Act of 1973. Rather, it concluded that the school's policy on requiring certification of medical fitness was appropriate and that the parents did not have the legal authority to waive their child's rights in these circumstances. Thus, the athlete was not judged to be otherwise qualified to participate (this athlete was cleared later to participate in college baseball at the University of Texas, Austin, after he signed a prospective release[27]).

Another, somewhat older case, *Poole v. South Plamfield Board of Education*, resulted in a different outcome.[13] In this case, a student with only one kidney was excluded from the varsity wrestling team by the school's medical officer. The plaintiff's parents found two outside physicians who offered medical judgments that the boy should be able to participate. The family brought a discrimination suit against the school, citing for support the provisions of the Rehabilitation Act of 1973. The court concluded that the plaintiff was qualified, except for his handicap, to participate in athletics since he met all the requirements and had opinions from two physicians to advocate clearance. The impression gained from a review of these and other cases suggests that the courts tend to consider the seriousness of a disorder and rely heavily on medical opinion before intervening to protect the athlete's rights under these federal laws or similar state statutes. In cases of cardiovascular abnormalities and serious risks in sports that impose intense cardiovascular demands, the courts likely would be reluctant to override medical decisions to exclude without at least one competent medical decision advocating clearance.

RECOMMENDATIONS FOR PHYSICIAN PRACTICE

Legal risk management reduces a practitioner's exposure to legal claim and suit and, in the event that suit is initiated, lessens the professional and financial consequences of an adverse outcome. In the practice of sports medicine, particularly with regard to screening and clearance activities for patients with cardiovascular disorders, a variety of approaches can be taken in the provision of service to manage legal risks. A frequently expressed concern is that legalistic thinking creates excessive documentation, threatens confidentiality, and interferes with the physician–patient relationship.[1] No risk management activities should be utilized that are excessively time-consuming. Justification for such activities in the health care setting comes from consideration of ethical responsibilities of the practitioner and the rights of patients to share fully in decisions affecting their own health and well-being. In reality, risk management activities that meet these criteria have the potential to enhance the physician–patient relationship and can be accomplished without excessive demands on the practitioner's time. The following activities deserve consideration by those engaged in clearing individuals with cardiovascular disorders for competitive sports:

1. Seek individualized advice from a local attorney to clarify, before the fact, the limits of legal responsibility that may affect the physician–patient relationship and confidentiality/disclosure requirements involving any third parties to whom the physician may be obliged to report. Communicate the conditions and limits of these provider responsibilities to the patient and, if appropriate, to family members and other third parties before agreeing to enter into the physician–patient relationship. Part of the legal consultation should involve examination and modification of any related documents that have a legal effect and that may be used in connection with delivery of services to adults or minor children, such as informed consent and permission forms for release of medical information to third parties (see the separate discussion of legal forms).
2. Reaffirm the relevance of medical guidelines and standards by which individual assessments and medical judgments are to be guided in these decisions to clear, prescribe limited activities, or exclude individuals from sports activities. Follow the most appropriate guidelines and protocols; annotate clinical records to document adherence; and, when deviation is indicated in the application of individual medical judgment, specify the reasons in the record with contemporaneous dated notes.
3. Communicate *in a timely way* with all parties to whom the physician has a duty and the authority to disclose any critical medical information or recommendations that may affect start, reentry, modification, discontinuation, or exclusion of a patient-athlete from a sports activity. Always document the timely conveyance of such critical communications.
4. Develop and use legally significant forms and procedures to support this process through consultation with an attorney and a risk manager. These may include forms for the informed consent process, authorization to release medical records/information, clearance or prohibition relative to sports participation, and, for certain situations, for express assumption of risk to document a disclaimer of responsibility for an athlete who enters competition against medical advice. Further explanation of this matter is presented in the following section.

Special Legal Forms

INFORMED CONSENT

Informed consent is a process whereby relevant information on a given medical procedure is provided to patients followed by an affirmative decision by the patient to undergo a particular treatment or procedure. In the sports medicine setting, litigation related to informed consent has focused on the claim that critical information was withheld, either negligently or intentionally, that was needed by the athlete to make an informed choice that every patient has a right to make. This is particularly problematic with elite amateur or professional athletes when a team physician may experience extreme pressure from coaches, the management, and even a player to allow clearance or reentry. In such situations, the practitioner should appreciate that these influences can exert subtle effects on judgment and lead to underappraisal of risk and/or understating the risk to the athlete, who depends greatly on the physician's judgment in these matters. The pressure to certify an individual as fit to compete[28] will always be a key issue in these circumstances. The informed consent process provides for an objective expression of these risks, a written record, and some evidence that the patient knew and understood the benefits, risks, and alternatives attendant on participating in any medical assessment or treatment. The duty of the physician to disclose information in the delivery of services is clear and has been substantiated repeatedly in judicial reviews. Physicians should be aware that the courts have been moving toward a requirement of broader and more detailed disclosure to patients of all foreseeable risks.[12]

RELEASES, WAIVERS, AND ASSUMPTIONS OF THE RISK

Many sports programs utilize written documents referred to as *releases, waivers,* or *assumptions of the risk*. Some practitioners use these forms to offset potential liability for untoward outcomes that may occur as a consequence of participation or medical treatment in connection with athletic situations. Comodeca, in recognition that waivers of liability have limited if any acceptable use in the medical setting, has suggested the possible risk management value of using an *acknowledgment of risk* statement within the informed consent document.[27]

In certain cases, prospective releases or similar documents may be used with some legal effect when athletes insist on participation despite medical advice to the contrary.[29,30] These situations arise most often in cases where the athlete has secured a second medical opinion that supports his or her clearance. These circumstances do create some difficulties because the process creates an avenue whereby some control for clearance decisions is shifted away from program personnel to outside parties. It must be pointed out, however, that these documents have been judged to be contrary to public policy in some circumstances in some states. Thus, their use may have no legal benefit in shielding programs, and particularly their physicians, from liability.[12]

There are numerous legal issues that have implications for the use of documents such as informed consent, waivers, prospective releases, and express assumptions of risk.[27,29–32] Extensive discussion can be found elsewhere, along with sample forms that have implications for use in the sports medicine setting.[33]

SUMMARY

1. Clearing athletes with cardiovascular disorders for athletic participation is a complex problem fraught with medical, ethical, and legal concerns. When confronted

with the need to examine, evaluate, and make recommendations about athletic participation in individuals with cardiovascular disorders, the physician often may face unreasonable expectations from the patient, family, and third parties who ascribe extraordinary importance to an affirmative decision. These circumstances challenge the physician ethically, complicate the traditional physician–patient relationship, and may create legal risks that are difficult to resolve.

2. Adherence to relevant practice guidelines affords a valuable approach to reducing the physician's risk. State statutes regulate the practice of medicine and provide a legal framework for examining the physician's performance in relation to relieving, curing, and safeguarding the health and well-being of patients. Claims of malpractice are often predicated on alleged failures of physician performance when compared to authoritative, widely accepted professional standards and guidelines. Courts and juries attempt to examine these claims through reference comparison of the physician's conduct against the standard, assessing whether any breach of the standard proximately caused the injury or death. Expert witness testimony often seeks to clarify proper application of the standard in court proceedings. Recommendations of the 26th Bethesda Conference[23] have cardinal importance in defining the legal standard of care for physician evaluation and medical eligibility decisions for athletes with cardiovascular abnormalities. Adherence to appropriate standards may be an effective shield against claim and suit, whereas injury or death that is proximately caused by failure to provide care according to the expected standards will render the physician liable.

   There is considerable variability among states in the laws that govern the practice of medicine. Federal statutes also exert certain influences. Ethical and legal obligations for confidentiality and disclosure of information by the physician may change depending on the physician's voluntary or remunerative role in the sports medicine setting and depending on whether they are attending a minor or an adult patient-athlete. The complexity of these circumstances clearly underscores the need for individualized legal consultation at the local level for any physician engaged in the practice of sports medicine, particularly when the responsibilities include critical recommendations about clearance of individuals with cardiovascular disorders.

3. Legal risk management seeks to inform patients more fully, preliminarily define practitioner duties in the physician–patient relationship, and utilize procedures/forms that may limit exposure to claim and suit. Effective risk management reduces the prospects of negligence findings and negative consequences arising from malpractice claims. In general, however, practicing under protocols that are sensitive to risk management issues has comprehensive and positive effects for both physicians and patients. Legally significant forms and risk management procedures should be developed through individualized consultation with an attorney and a risk manager.

REFERENCES

1. Macri PA: The negative effect of the legal system on sports medicine. *Sports Med Standards Malpractice Rep* 6:1, 3–5, 1994.

2. Maron BJ: Sudden death in young athletes: Lessons from the Hank Gathers affair. *N Engl J Med* 329:55–57, 1993.
3. Van Camp SP, Bloor CM, Mueller FO, et al: Nontraumatic sports death in high school and college athletes. *Med Sci Sports Exerc* 27:641–647, 1995.
4. Mitchell JH, Haskell WL, Raven PB: Classification of sports. *Med Sci Sports Exerc* 26:S242–S245, 1995.
5. Maron BJ, Brown RW, McGrew CA, et al: Ethical, legal, and practical considerations impacting medical decision-making in competitive athletes. *Med Sci Sports Exerc* 26:S230–S237, 1995.
6. Macri PA: Returning athletes for play: The physician's perspective. *Sports Med Standards Malpractice Rep* 6:53–54, 1994.
7. Murray TH: Divided loyalties in sports medicine. *Phys Sportsmed* 12:134–140, 1984.
8. McKeag DB, Brody H, Hough DO: Medical ethics in sport. *Phys Sportsmed* 12:145–148, 150, 1984.
9. Herbert DL: The death of Hank Gathers: An examination of the legal issues. *Sports Med Standards Malpractice Rep* 2:45–47, 1990.
10. Gallup E: Death on the court: A look at the tragic death of NBA star Reggie Lewis. *Sports Med Standards Malpractice Rep* 6:12, 1994.
11. Herbert DL: Sports medicine team duties and responsibilities. In Herbert DL, Herbert WG: *Legal Aspects of Sports Medicine.* Canton, Ohio, Professional Reports Corporation, 1990, pp 169–173.
12. Herbert DL, Herbert WG: Medical-legal issues. In Cantu RC, Micheli LJ (eds): *ACSM's Guidelines for the Team Physician*. Philadelphia, Lea and Febiger, 1991, pp 119–126.
13. Herbert DL: Sports medicine team duties and responsibilities. In Herbert DL, Herbert WG: *Legal Aspects of Sports Medicine.* Canton, Ohio, Professional Reports Corporation, 1990, pp 13–21.
14. Herbert DL: New subspecialty created. *Sports Med Standards Malpractice Rep* 5:37, 1993.
15. Herbert DL: Statutory volunteer immunity for sports medicine practitioners. *Sports Med Standards Malpractice Rep* 4:10–11, 1992.
16. Editorial: Year end review: Medicine by the book. *Am Med News* 1:28, 1989.
17. Herbert DL: Should sports medicine providers rely on practice parameters? *Sports Med Standards Malpractice Rep* 7:25–26, 1995.
18. Hyams AL, Brandenburg JA, Lipsitz SR, et al: Practice guidelines and malpractice litigation: A two-way street. *Ann Intern Med* 122:450–455, 1995.
19. American College of Sports Medicine: *Guidelines for Exercise Testing and Exercise Prescription*, ed 4. Philadelphia, Lea and Febiger, 1991.
20. Joint Task Force on Assessment of Cardiovascular Procedures, the American College of Cardiology/American Heart Association: Special report: Guidelines for exercise testing. *Circulation* 74:653A–667A, 1986.
21. Committee on Competitive Safeguards and Medical Aspects of Sports, National Collegiate Athletic Association: *Sports Medicine Handbook,* ed 3. Mission, Kan, NCAA, 1988.
22. Committee on Sports Medicine, American Academy of Pediatrics: Recommendations for participation in competitive sports. *Pediatrics* 81:737–739, 1988.
23. The 26th Bethesda Conference: Recommendations for determining eligibility for competition in athletes with cardiovascular abnormalities. *Med Sci Sports Exerc* 26 (Suppl):S223–S283, 1994.
24. Maron BJ, Mitchell JH: Revised eligibility recommendations for competitive athletes with cardiovascular abnormalities. *Med Sci Sports Exerc* 26:S223–S225, 1995.
25. Mitten MJ, and Maron BJ: Legal considerations that affect medical eligibility for competitive athletes with cardiovascular abnormalities and acceptance of Bethesda Conference recommendations. *Med Sci Sports Exerc* 26:S238–S241, 1995.

26. Graham TP, Bricker JT, James FW, et al: Congenital heart disease. *Med Sci Sports Exerc* 26:S246–S253, 1995.
27. Comodeca JA: Acknowledgment of risk forms: The best defense for sports medicine practitioners. *Sports Med Standards Malpractice Rep* 4:49, 51–54, 1992.
28. Leslie CG: War and peace with Hippocrates—a modern dilemma facing sports medicine. *Sports Med Standards Malpractice Rep* 2:21, 24–28, 1990.
29. Herbert DL: Prospective releases: Will their use protect sports medicine physicians from suit? *Sports Med Standards Malpractice Rep* 6:33, 35–36, 1994.
30. Herbert DL: Express assumption of risk and decisions to exclude from play—the sports medicine dilemma. *Sports Med Standards Malpractice Rep* 2:1, 3–7, 1990.
31. Sahlin JH: Letter to the editor: McCorkle v. Hall: Exculpatory clauses. *Sports Med Standards Malpractice Rep* 2:78–79, 1990.
32. Herbert DL: Word choices for informed consent documents may render process invalid. *Sports Med Standards Malpractice Rep* 4:40–41, 1992.
33. Herbert DL: Sample forms and documents. In Herbert DL, Herbert WG (eds): *Legal Aspects of Sports Medicine.* Canton, Ohio, Professional Reports Corporation, 1990, pp 261–296.

APPENDICES

APPENDIX 1. Classification of sports activities by levels of dynamic and static demands

	A. Low Dynamic	B. Moderate Dynamic	C. High Dynamic
I. Low static	Billiards Bowling Golf	Baseball Softball Table tennis Tennis, doubles Volleyball	Badminton Cross-country skiing, classic style Racquetball Running, long-distance Soccer* Tennis, singles
II. Moderate static	Archery Diving*† Equestrian*†	Fencing Figure skating* Football* Rugby* Running, sprinting Surfing*†	Basketball* Ice hockey* Cross-country skiing, skating style Lacrosse* Swimming
III. High static	Bobsledding*† Gymnastics*† Karate/judo* Rock climbing*† Sailing Water skiing*† Weight lifting*†	Downhill skiing*† Wrestling*	Boxing* Canoeing/kayaking Cycling*† Rowing Speed skating

*Risk of body collision.

†High risk for patients prone to syncope.

Source: Adapted with permission from Mitchell JH, Haskell WL, Raven PB. Classification of sports. *Med Sci Sports Exerc* 26(Suppl):S242–S245, 1994.

APPENDIX 2. Caloric demands of physical activities

Activity	Intensity	Energy Demands (METS)
Archery	Nonhunting	3.5
Badminton	Competitive	7.0
	Leisure	4.5
Baseball	General	5.0
Basketball	Game	8.0
	Shooting baskets	4.5
Bicycling	Leisure, light effort, <10 mph	4.0
	Leisure, moderate effort, 12–14 mph	8.0
	Stationary, general	5.0
Billiards	General	2.5
Bobsledding	General	7.0
Bowling	General	3.0
Boxing	General	12.0
Canoeing/kayaking	Rowing, moderate effort, 4–6 mph	7.0
Diving	Springboard or platform	3.0
Equestrian	General	4.0
Fencing	General	6.0
Football	Competitive	9.0
	Noncompetitive, general	8.0
Golf	General	4.5
Gymnastics	General	4.0
Ice hockey	General	8.0
Inactive, resting	Sitting quietly	1.0
Karate/judo	General	10.0
Lacrosse	General	8.0
Racquetball	Competitive	10.0
	Casual, general	7.0
Rock climbing	Ascending	11.0
	Rapelling	8.0
Rugby	General	10.0
Running	Long distance	9.0
	Intermediate distance/effort, 6 mph	10.0
	Sprints	16.0
Sailing	General	3.0
Skating	Ice, general	7.0
Ice, figure	Ice, figure skating	9.0
Roller	Roller skating	7.0
Skiing	Cross-country, classic, moderate effort	8.0
	Cross-country, skating, moderate effort	9.0
	Downhill, moderate effort	6.0
	Water skiing	6.0
Soccer	Competitive	10.0
	Noncompetitive, general	7.0
Softball	General	5.0

APPENDIX 2. ***Continued***

Activity	Intensity	Energy Demands (METS)
Swimming	Leisurely, general	6.0
	Swimming laps, vigorous effort, freestyle	10.0
	Backstroke, general	8.0
	Breaststroke, general	10.0
	Butterfly, general	11.0
Surfing	Body or board	3.0
Tennis	Lawn, doubles	6.0
	Lawn, singles	8.0
	Table tennis (ping-pong)	4.0
Volleyball	Competitive	4.0
	Noncompetitive, general	3.0
	Beach	8.0
Weight lifting	Light to moderate	3.0

Source: Adapted with permission from Ainsworth BE, Haskell WL, Leon AS, et al: Compendium of physical activities: Classification of energy costs of human physical activities. *Med Sci Sports Exerc* 25:71–80, 1993.

INDEX

Italics refer to figures
t refers to tables.

Q

R

S